COUNTRY DOCTOR'S
=== BOOK OF ===
MEDICAL WISDOM
AND CURES

MICHAEL J. CUMMINGS

CONSULTANT: B. TED BOADWAY, M.D.

PUBLICATIONS INTERNATIONAL, LTD.

Notice:
In this book, the author, consultant, and editors have done their best to outline the symptoms and general treatment for various conditions, injuries, and diseases. Also, recommendations are made regarding certain drugs, medications, and preparations; and descriptions of certain medical tests and procedures are offered. Different people react to the same treatment, medication, preparation, test, or procedure in different ways. This book does not attempt to answer all questions about all situations that you may encounter.

Neither the Editors of Consumer Guide® and Publications International, Ltd., nor the consultants, authors, or publisher take responsibility for any possible consequence from any treatment, procedure, test, action, or application of medication or preparation by any person reading or following the information in this book. The publication of this book does not constitute the practice of medicine, and this book does not attempt to replace your physician. The contributors and the publisher advise the reader to check with a physician before administering any medication or undertaking any course of treatment.

Michael J. Cummings is the author of dozens of health-related articles for various newspapers, magazines, and medical publications. He is a former managing editor of *Grit* and a frequent contributor to *Hospital Benchmarks, Geisinger Medical Center Magazine,* and *FDA Consumer.* Mr. Cummings serves as an adjunct writing instructor at the Pennsylvania College of Technology in Williamsport, Pennsylvania.

B. Ted Boadway, M.D., spent 13 years as a family physician in Thornhill, outside of Toronto, before joining the staff of the Ontario Medical Association, where he currently serves as executive director of the Department of Health Policy. He earned his medical degree at the University of Toronto and is a former medical director of Extendicare North York, a 300-bed chronic-care facility. For more than 11 years, Dr. Boadway has been heard regularly on Canadian Broadcasting Corporation national radio programs. He is the author of *Chicken Soup and Other Nostrums.*

Cover Illustration: Robert Crawford

Illustrations: Steven Noble

ISBN: 0-7853-2307-4

CONTENTS

AT-HOME HEALING

Got a backache? Are you tense or depressed? What's the best way to treat a bee sting, a sunburn, or an earache? *Country Doctor's Book of Medical Wisdom and Cures* offers doctor-approved lifestyle strategies and timeless home remedies you can use safely and effectively—for everything from colds and constipation to urinary tract infections and warts.

If you're among those who smoke, if you drink too much, eat a diet high in fat, or succumb too readily to the comforts of an easy chair, you are declaring yourself open prey for the great killer afflictions of our time: heart disease and cancer. If you need to walk away from an unhealthy lifestyle—and leave behind a trail of bad habits—use this book to form the foundation on which to build your wellness program. You'll find sensible advice about nutrition, exercise, stress reduction, addiction avoidance, and coping with depression. Follow these words of wisdom and you'll be taking an important step toward gaining control of your lifestyle and making the right health choices.

Country Doctor's Book of Medical Wisdom and Cures offers many tried-and-true therapies, including herbal remedies that can be used to treat a migraine, soothe a cold, and fight infection. Some of these homespun remedies require little preparation—like cranberry juice, which, according to research, may be effective in preventing bladder infections. Others—such as the yarrow poultice that helps heal minor cuts and abrasions—will require more effort. You will need to combine powders or oils with other ingredients before using them.

Like prescription medications, these home remedies may work well for some people and not so well for others. If a particular remedy doesn't seem right for you, check with your doctor before using it—or simply don't use it at all.

Be aware that you should not attempt to treat serious illnesses—or suspected serious illnesses—with the home remedies discussed in this book without first consulting a doctor. Self-treatment may only delay the professional treatment you require and, if the illness worsens, diminish your chances for complete and quick recovery.

As you use *Country Doctor's Book of Medical Wisdom and Cures,* share the information with members of your family, especially those who could most benefit by it, such as smokers and couch potatoes. Perhaps you'll even decide to launch a wellness program together.

Remember, folks, there is strength in numbers.

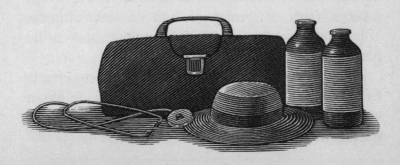

LIVING WELL

"Habit is habit," Mark Twain wrote, "and not to be flung out the window by any man, but coaxed downstairs a step at a time."

Now is the time to gather up your bad habits, coax them downstairs, and send them packing. More than any medication or hospital machine, it is your lifestyle that plays the biggest role in whether you stay well. Unfortunately, a good many folks refuse to accept that fact.

According to the National Institutes of Health, half of all Americans don't get regular exercise. Eighty percent refuse to eat the right foods. One-third of adults and nearly one-fifth of children are overweight. And sixty million Americans—both young and old—continue to smoke cigarettes.

Obviously these folks need a good talking to. Afflictions caused by unhealthy lifestyles include high blood pressure, heart disease, stroke, lung cancer, emphysema, obesity, cirrhosis of the liver, stress, and depression. It isn't easy to overcome old habits. What it takes is grit, determination, and a positive attitude. You must want to be well. You must choose to be healthy.

This chapter will assist you in your wellness efforts by providing useful information and advice about smoking, alcohol abuse, nutrition, exercise, and stress management.

SMOKING AND ALCOHOL ABUSE

According to author Alvin Schwartz, there was once a town so healthy they had to shoot somebody to start a cemetery.

It's a safe bet that nobody in that town—wherever it was—drank to excess or smoked cigarettes. Smoking and drinking are, after all, the twin terrors of medicine. In terms of illness, family problems, lost work days, social discord, and death by accident, disease, and suicide, these vices rival the devastation of an all-out war. In fact, cigarettes and alcohol have killed more Americans—dentists, barbers, bellboys, plumbers, waitresses, farmers—than all the wars in America since Columbus' arrival.

Cigarettes alone figure in the deaths of nearly 400,000 Americans every year and in the illness of millions more. (If you tend to prefer comparisons, that would be like having the entire population of North and South Dakota die every three years.) And no wonder. Among the approximately 300 known poisons in tobacco smoke are arsenic, cyanide, carbon monoxide, and formaldehyde.

Practically everyone knows that cigarettes cause lung cancer. But not everyone is aware that cigarettes also cause cancer of the mouth, larynx, esophagus, stomach, bladder, kidney, blood, and pancreas. Cigarettes also cause high blood pressure, heart disease, stroke, emphysema, and chronic bronchitis. According to research from the Rose Medical Center in Denver, Colorado, a 25-year-old who smokes two packs of cigarettes a day will die 8.3 years sooner than a nonsmoker. Think of what those 8.3 years mean: all the unwritten letters, the unattended family reunions, and the unspoken conversations with your children and grandchildren.

But the devastation doesn't end with the smoker. Nonsmokers exposed to secondary smoke at home or at work can develop thickening of the arteries ten percent faster than unexposed nonsmokers, according to a study of 8,415 people by the Bowman Gray School of Medicine in Winston-Salem, North Carolina. Children of smokers are among the most frequent victims of secondary smoke: They suffer more respiratory problems and miss more school days than children of nonsmokers.

Another hazard to society's well-being is the bottle. Alcohol abuse is a major cause of violence, suicide, economic ruin, and family turmoil. It contributes to the deaths of 100,000 Americans every year from alcohol-related forms of cancer, heart disease, liver disease, and other illnesses. In addition, alcohol kills or injures thousands more in alcohol-related motor-vehicle accidents. An organization called Mothers Against Drunk Driving (MADD) provides some grim statistics:

Some 16,589 persons died in alcohol-related traffic accidents in 1994, accounting for 40.8 percent of all traffic fatalities. In that same year, one million people suffered injuries in alcohol-related traffic accidents. Two of every five Americans will be involved in an alcohol-related motor-vehicle accident at some time in their lives unless remedial action is taken.

If you're among those who smoke cigarettes or drink alcohol to excess, tell your physician. Your doctor can support and advise you as you struggle with your habit—and point you in the right direction when you decide to give it up. The good news is that quitting your habit can instantly improve your well-being. In many cases, your body immediately begins to repair the damage that has been done: Within 15 years, an ex-smoker's risk of suffering a heart attack will be about the same as a nonsmoker's.

No, quitting is not easy. But it is well within everyone's capability, as millions of former smokers and problem drinkers have proven. Begin by admitting you have a problem. Then—with the assistance of relatives, friends, and your physician—determine why you continue to support your bad habits. For example, do you smoke or drink to relieve tension? If so, ask yourself what's causing the tension. Tight deadlines at work? Money problems? Feelings of social inadequacy? (Many people light up cigarettes in so-

A WEIGHTY ISSUE

If you are attempting to quit smoking, you may be worried about gaining weight. Although you may gain five to ten pounds initially, quitting smoking greatly reduces the likelihood of suffering from lung cancer and chronic lung diseases down the road. The American Lung Association offers these tips to help you in your struggle to stop smoking and keep weight gain to a minimum:

- Recognize that it will be more difficult to quit smoking if you focus on dieting at the same time. You can design a healthy plan for losing weight after you quit.
- Incorporate an exercise regimen into your daily activities. Exercise can be used as a potential substitute activity to distract you from the urge to smoke.
- Adhere to a healthy, nutritional weight-control plan.

cial situations to have "something to do with their hands." Some people drink to excess to lower their inhibitions.)

Once you know what's behind your habit, you can begin working on eliminating its cause. When properly motivated, some smokers can quit cold turkey. Others find it helpful to join a support group, seek counseling, or enroll in a smoking-cessation program.

University of Texas researchers have found that "scheduled smoking" can help people quit. Here's how it works: When cutting down, you decide to smoke only at certain times—say 8 A.M., 2 P.M., and 8 P.M. In doing so, you reduce the effects of subtle smoking prompts such as coffee, food, stress, and fatigue. Eventually the prompts lose their effect, making it easier to quit smoking altogether. One year after a scheduled-smoking study, researchers said 44 percent of the people who "quit by the clock" remained non-smokers, compared with 22 percent who quit cold-turkey and 18 percent who quit in other ways.

One aid that has come along in recent years is the transdermal nicotine patch, now available at drugstores without a doctor's prescription. This device is a tiny decal the user sticks to the skin. During the day the patch releases nicotine into the body, satisfying the smoker's physical need for the drug. Over a period of weeks or months, the dosage released gradually declines, weaning the user off nicotine. Studies have shown that the success rate of the transdermal nico-

CIGAR, ANYONE?

Is cigar smoking safe? The American Lung Association offers the following response to some common myths:

Myth: Cigar smoking is a safe alternative to cigarettes.

Fact: Cigar smokers are four to ten times more likely to die from laryngeal, oral, and esophageal cancers than nonsmokers.

Myth: Cigars aren't addictive.

Fact: Cigars, like cigarettes, contain nicotine, a highly addictive substance.

Myth: Cigar smoking doesn't cause lung diseases because you don't inhale.

Fact: While the risk of lung cancer is lower for cigar smokers than cigarette smokers, the risk increases with more frequent cigar smoking. In fact, men who smoke at least five cigars a day are two to three times more likely to die of lung cancer than nonsmokers.

tine patch doubles when the user couples the program with participation in a support group.

Unfortunately, there's no "alcohol patch" for problem drinkers. And cutting down gradually on your own just won't work, because one small portion of alcohol inevitably leads to another—and another, and another.

If you're a short-term problem drinker, you may not require hospitalization or other extraordinary measures, but you surely will need the help of others. Many problem drinkers have found the organization Alcoholics Anonymous to be a very effective program. (AA members include not only short-term problem drinkers but also alcoholics who have "dried out" at detoxification clinics.) At AA meetings, alcohol abusers share their experiences and receive psychological support. Through AA's famous Twelve Step program, members learn to abstain one day at a time. There are no fees. There are no special requirements to join.

Drugs are also available to help ease the transition to sobriety. One of them, Antabuse, makes you sick whenever you drink. Other drugs make the effects of alcohol less pronounced and, therefore, less pleasurable.

If an underlying psychological problem caused you to begin drinking in the first place, or if a psychological problem arose while you were drinking, you may also need to undergo counseling as you adjust to your new, healthier lifestyle.

(Recognizing that alcohol abuse is a problem for the people around the drinker, not just the drinker alone,

AA also operates Al-Anon for family members and Alateen for teenage children of alcoholics. In such groups relatives not only learn how to cope in their environment, but they can also learn how to support the alcoholic during the difficult recovery period.)

Once you kick your addiction you will experience an urge to resume your habit from time to time. But those feelings will lessen over time as new, more productive activities occupy your energies, and new routines and patterns replace the old.

EATING WELL

One day experts say milk is good for you because it contains calcium and builds strong bones. The next day they say milk is bad for you because it contains artery-clogging saturated fat. Who do you believe?

There's probably a little bit of truth in much of what you read and hear. But there's a lot of truth in what the Greeks advised centuries ago: "All things in moderation, nothing in excess." To that, we should add the following commonsense principles:

1. Tailor your daily diet to your medical history.

No two people are the same. Their blood pressure, cholesterol level, and metabolic

FISH OIL

A study conducted by the University of Washington found that people who ate three ounces of salmon a week reduced their risk of cardiac arrest by 50 percent.

Researchers theorize that omega-3 fatty acids in salmon and other fish appear to enhance the electrical activity in the heart. Besides reducing the risk of cardiac arrest, the fatty acids, which are found in fish oil, may also lower the risk of other forms of heart disease.

The American Heart Association recommends that Americans regularly include fish in their diet. However, many experts caution against the use of fish-oil supplements. Some supplements contain vitamins that could be toxic when taken in high doses.

SPINACH AND OLDER EYES

Spinach may help prevent vision loss in the elderly. Ophthalmologist Johanna Seddon, M.D., of the Massachusetts Eye and Ear Infirmary in Boston, reached that conclusion after she and researchers at five other institutions studied the eating habits of 876 patients. The study found that the more fruits and vegetables you eat—particularly spinach and collard greens—the less likely you'll be to develop macular degeneration. Macular degeneration involves cell death and leakage of blood vessels in the eye, a condition that can lead to blindness.

Dietary measures, of course, can't treat macular degeneration. Only physicians can do that. But eating plenty of fruits and vegetables can help prevent macular degeneration from developing in the first place.

rate differ. Therefore, because you are different, it's best to learn all you can about your body before you develop a plan to improve your diet. If a physical exam reveals you have high blood pressure, for example, you will have to cut down on salty foods and remove the salt shaker from the table. If you're allergic to milk, which is rich in calcium, you'll have to place other calcium-rich foods on your menu. If you're frequently tense or anxious, you may have to avoid caffeinated products. Talk with your physician. The more you know about your nutritional needs, the better you will be able to fulfill them.

2. Eat a variety of foods.

From time to time, most of us indulge in a hearty meal of meat and potatoes. But if you eat meat and potatoes every noon and night, you won't get the variety of nutrients your body needs. Eventually you could develop a nutritional deficiency that could lead to illness. For example, a calcium deficiency can result in the bone-weakening disease osteoporosis. Iron deficiency can lead to the fatiguing condition known as anemia. And a deficiency in B-complex vitamins can lead to nerve disorders and nausea. Some of the more than 100 symptoms or conditions caused by or associated with vitamin and mineral deficiencies include muscle weakness, insomnia, depression, diarrhea, constipation, dizziness, headache, apathy, dry skin, itching, trembling, numbness, irritability, and loss of appetite.

Which foods should you eat and in what amounts?

First, make fruits, vegetables, grains, and legumes the mainstay of your diet, accounting for 55 to 60 percent of your total calorie intake. In its dietary guidelines, the U.S Department of Agriculture (USDA) recommends that you eat 6 to 11 servings of grain products a day, 3 to 5 servings of vegetables and legumes, and 2 to 4 servings of fruit. These foods are generally very low in fat and very high in essential nutrients. Besides providing the vitamins, minerals, amino acids, and other nutrients you need to remain healthy, these foods are also an excellent source of fiber, or roughage. This coarse, stringy substance not only helps cleanse your body of excess fat and cholesterol and promotes regular bowel movements, but it also appears to reduce your risk of developing colon cancer and other intestinal diseases. An excellent source of fiber is breakfast cereal; look for the fiber content listing on the side of the box. Salads, vegetables, and whole-grain breads are also good sources of fiber.

Second, eat moderate amounts of foods in the meat group (red meat, poultry, fish, eggs, and nuts) and the milk group (milk, cheese, yogurt, and other dairy products). According to the USDA, two to three servings a day from each group will meet your nutritional needs. Moderation is necessary because many foods in these groups contain high amounts of saturated fat and cholesterol, which can contribute to the development of heart disease and other illnesses. (A diet high in saturated fats—including those animal fats found in butter and meats—has been found to increase the serum cholesterol level in the blood and, therefore, increase the risk of developing atherosclerosis. Less-saturated fats, such as those found in olive oil, canola oil, and the oils in some fish and nuts, are better dietary choices.)

Although the foods found in both the meat and milk groups are excellent sources of protein—which is vital to building and maintaining organs, muscles, cartilage, and skin—your body doesn't require large amounts of protein. According to standards set by the Food and Nutrition Board of the National Academy of Sciences, a 150-pound person requires about 66 grams of protein a day. A four-ounce hamburger alone will meet half that requirement. What if you eat more protein than you need? If you're healthy, the extra protein will probably be converted to sugar. It's the saturated fat and cholesterol found in most protein-containing foods that should concern you—they may remain in the body as excess fat, potentially causing serious health problems.

3. Eat only the number of calories your body really needs.

It's not how many calories you consume that matters. It's whether you use those calories. If you're an

Olympic swimmer, a lumberjack, or a letter carrier, you require more calories than the average person because you expend more calories. It's simple arithmetic. However, if you take in 3,500 calories a day but use only 2,500, your body will store the extra calories as fat. If you make a habit of piling up fat, you'll gain weight. And if you exceed your recommended weight by 20 or 30 pounds—that is, if you become obese—you'll increase your risk of developing a range of diseases. In recent years, Americans have, in fact, been piling up fat. According to the USDA, between 1991 and 1994 the average American gained 11 pounds.

Obesity is the leading cause of diabetes in the United States, according to Michael D. Myers, M.D., a specialist in eating and weight disorders in Los Alamitos, California. But the risks don't stop there. Obesity can also significantly increase the risk of developing high blood pressure, heart disease, degenerative arthritis, gallstones, and cancer. And, Myers says, obese women may have triple the risk of developing cancer of the breast, uterus, cervix, and ovaries.

So how many calories does the average person need? Victor Herbert, M.D., a professor at the Mount Sinai School of Medicine in New York, says an average "sedentary adult" requires about 10 calories for each pound of weight to perform basic functions such as breathing, digesting food, and circulating blood. In addition, this sedentary adult requires 3 calories for each pound of weight to carry out routine daily activities, such as walking, eating, or driving a car. Thus, a 175-pound sedentary man would need 2,275 calories a day (175×10 plus 175×3). If this man decided to take up tennis, expending an additional 500 calories each day, then he would need 2,775 calories a day (2,275 plus 500).

4. Limit your intake of fat.

Fat makes food taste good. And a certain amount of it is essential to provide energy and enable the body to absorb vitamins A, D, E, and K. You will find an abundance of fat in sausage, most red meats, bacon, salad dressings, deep-fried battered foods, potato chips, ice cream—practically anything that's greasy or creamy. Unfortunately, fat promotes weight gain. (One gram of fat contains 9 calories; one gram of protein or carbohydrates contains only 4 calories). And weight gain can lead to a variety of serious health problems.

The worst kind of fat is saturated fat. It causes the body to produce excessive amounts of cholesterol. Cholesterol that's deposited in your arteries is known as plaque. Over time, these plaques may grow larger and larger. Blood platelets that circulate through your body to aid in clotting sometimes stick to plaque deposits, making them grow all the faster. Eventually, a plaque deposit can grow so large that it cuts off the flow of blood and its life-giving oxygen. When that happens, you could suffer a heart attack or stroke. As a rule, try to stick with foods that are low in saturated fat. Generally, no more than 30 percent of your calories should come from fats, and no more than 10 percent should come from saturated fats.

5. Limit your cholesterol intake.

Cholesterol helps your body produce bile acids, cell membranes, sex hormones, and the protective covering of nerves called myelin. Interestingly, your body produces just about all the cholesterol it needs. Therefore, the cholesterol you get from food is overkill. And if you continually overload your body with cholesterol, you put your arteries at risk of becoming clogged with plaque. Among the foods high in cholesterol are organ meats, eggs, desserts, and many of the foods that are high in saturated fat. As a general rule, you should limit your intake of cholesterol to no more than 300 milligrams a day.

6. Go easy on salt.

Salt consists of 40 percent sodium and 60 percent chloride. The sodium in salt is vital to maintaining your body's fluid balance and blood pressure. You couldn't live without sodium. The trouble is, as with cholesterol, a little bit of sodium goes a long way. In fact, you need only about 500 milligrams of sodium a day, roughly the amount contained in one-fifth of a teaspoon of salt.

The maximum intake of sodium should not exceed 2,400 milligrams a day, or about a teaspoon of salt, according to U.S. government guidelines. Among foods high in sodium content are bacon, ham, smoked fish, corned beef, pickles, olives, frozen dinners, salad dressings, and practically all canned and processed foods. (Fresh foods usually contain little or no sodium.)

To monitor your sodium intake, read disclosure labels on cartons, packages, and cans, then mark down the amount of sodium you consume when you eat a serving of food. For example, if you eat a serving of bean soup for lunch, you would mark down the amount of 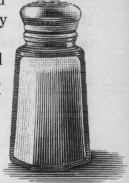 sodium in one serving—about 800 milligrams. That would mean you could consume 1,600 more milligrams of sodium during the day before reaching the maximum recommended intake of 2,400 milligrams.

7. Go easy on sugar.

Table sugar, or sucrose, is only one of many kinds of sugar. Other varieties occur naturally in foods. The sugar lactose occurs in milk, and the sugar maltose occurs in the malt in beer. Fruit contains a very sweet sugar called fructose; it also contains the sugars sucrose and glucose.

Your body manufactures glucose from the fruit, vegetables, grains, and other carbohydrates you eat. Glucose is important to the body because it provides fuel and maintains the proper functioning of cells. However, because the body can make or acquire all the glucose it needs from natural foods, you don't need to add glucose—or any other kinds of sugars—to the foods you eat.

KEEPING FIT

When Anne Clarke, of Carol Stream, Illinois, ran a series of footraces in the late 1980s, she sometimes had to compete against younger runners—people who were in their sixties or early seventies. "But I still managed to win 40 national awards," she said. She turned 80 in 1989.

Clarke, a retired teacher, would run five to seven miles a day to stay fit and to train for local, national, and international events, including 10-kilometer races. No doubt some interested onlookers may have wondered if that sort of vigorous exercise was really safe for folks her age.

The fact is, everyone in every age group who is generally healthy and physically able should exercise vigorously—and often. Karl F. Hempel, M.D., a family physician in Tallahassee, Florida, and a diplomate of the American Board of Family Practice, says, according to new government guidelines, everyone should exercise at least 30 minutes a day seven days a week. (But the daily exercise can be cumulative: Two 15-minute exercise periods—or three 10-minute periods—will meet the day's recommended 30-minute requirement.)

What's so good about exercise? Well, besides enabling you to run races, it also:

- Lowers your blood pressure if it is already too high
- Reduces the risk of developing high blood pressure down the road

DRINK UP

Whether you are jogging or biking around the neighborhood or scaling Mt. Everest, make sure you are well hydrated. Drink at least two cups of fluid two hours before you even begin to work out. Also, plan to drink at least a half cup of water every 20 minutes while you exercise. After exercise, don't forget to replace fluids: Approximately two cups of water for every pound of fluid you lost.

Replacing fluids lost to sweat is the number-one rule for any exerciser. And, contrary to what advertisers would have you believe, drinking plain water is the best way to put back fluids you've lost.

When exercising, remember to watch for early signs of dehydration: fatigue, flushed skin, heat intolerance, light-headedness, and dark urine with a strong odor.

Living Well

- Decreases your risk of developing heart disease and improves your survivability if you have heart disease
- Enables you to control your weight
- Strengthens your muscles
- Maintains your bone density
- Reduces tension and anxiety
- Improves your physical appearance

Must you run races or climb mountains to stay in shape? Not at all. Americans who don't regularly exercise can achieve cardiovascular fitness simply by walking, riding a bike, or even dancing. Cardiovascular fitness refers to the body's ability to deliver and process oxygen at optimum levels. In other words, if you are cardiovascularly fit, your heart will pump more oxygen per beat, and you will have more endurance. With regular vigorous exercise, your heart will become stronger and stronger, and it will be able to meet demands more efficiently.

Activities that build cardiovascular fitness are called aerobic exercises because they cause sustained heavy breathing. Swimming, skiing, and skipping rope are all

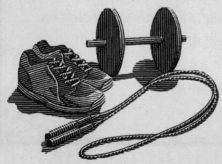

aerobic activities. If you regularly exercise aerobically, you can achieve a high level of cardiovascular fitness. Activities that keep you in motion produce better

In the Beginning

For your health's sake, always check with your doctor before you embark on a new exercise program, especially if you answer "yes" to any of the following questions:

1. Has my doctor ever told me I have heart disease?
2. Do I suffer from chest pains?
3. Has my doctor said that my blood pressure is too high?
4. Has my doctor told me that I have a bone or joint problem, such as arthritis?
5. Am I overweight?
6. Have I avoided exercising on a regular basis?
7. Am I taking prescription medications, such as those for high blood pressure?
8. Is there any reason why I shouldn't begin an exercise program?

results than activities that make you stop and start repeatedly. For example, although playing golf is good exercise, it does not require a long period of sustained exertion. You walk, then stop; you walk, then stop. Jogging and roller-skating, on the other hand, keep you moving constantly, giving your heart a good workout. (There are also some good old-fashioned exercises that can boost cardiovascular fitness, including pitching hay, pulling weeds, and digging post holes. Just don't stop to gossip with the neighbors for too long.)

Besides aerobic exercise, it's a good idea to include in your regimen exercises that increase muscle strength and flexibility. The stronger and more flexible you are, the less likely you will be to pull a muscle, tear a ligament, throw out your back, or break a bone. Push-ups are an excellent exercise to improve upper body strength. And stretching exercises will increase your overall muscle elasticity, enabling you to bend, turn, and pivot with less risk of injury.

Before you start a vigorous exercise program, you should have a physical exam. For middle-aged and older folks, this examination should include a stress test designed to detect heart problems. The test is relatively simple. While you walk or run on a treadmill, monitors attached to your chest measure your heart activity as well as your blood pressure and pulse.

After receiving your physician's okay, choose one or more activities you are likely to enjoy and stick with them. If they require special equipment—such as running shoes for jogging or a protective helmet for biking—be sure to select comfortable, high-quality products.

Precede each of your workouts with a warm-up period that gradually elevates the heart rate and increases the flow of oxygen-rich blood to the muscles. Five to ten minutes of moderate activity, such as stretching your arms and your legs, is usually a sufficient warm-up period.

At the end of your workout, don't stop abruptly. Instead, cool down by gradually slowing your activity. Cooldowns help prevent a sudden drop in blood pressure. Moreover, they reduce the likelihood that you will become stiff and sore after your workout.

During the first few weeks of your exercise program, don't try to reach all of your exercise goals at once. Instead, break yourself in gradually. For example, if brisk walking is your choice of exercise, you might consider limiting yourself to a half-mile or so early on, then increasing your distance to a mile and beyond. Trying to accomplish workout goals too quickly can result in serious injury: Remember, you're in it for the long haul. If at any time you sense that you are overtaxing yourself, it's probably a sign you *are* trying to do too much too soon. If exercise causes chest pain, faintness, dizziness, or weakness, or it causes you to gasp for air, stop your activity immediately and pay a visit to your physician.

ADVICE FOR LIFE

The National Cancer Institute offers the following suggestions on making your life a whole lot healthier:

- Don't use tobacco. If you do, quit.
- Eat at least five servings of fruits and vegetables each day. Fruits and vegetables may lower your risk for some kinds of cancer.
- If you are a woman age 50 or older, get a mammogram every one to two years.
- Every woman—even those who have gone through menopause—should have regular checkups that include a pelvic exam and a Pap test.
- Cancers of the colon, rectum, and prostate are more likely to occur in the elderly. Ask your doctor how often you should be tested for these conditions.
- Avoid too much sunlight and wear protective clothing and sunscreen when outdoors.

If you live in an area where severe weather conditions keep you indoors in the winter or summer, consider investing in exercise equipment, such as treadmills, rowing machines, aerobic riders, and exercise bikes. The more sophisticated machines can monitor your heart rate and keep a daily record of your activities. Of course, you can turn the weather to your advantage, too. In the winter, you can ski or ice-skate. In the summer, try swimming or go canoeing.

Whatever exercise you do, the important thing is to keep doing it. Continuing your exercise program will help you live a longer, healthier life.

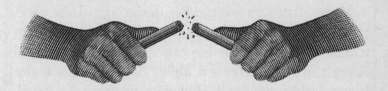

MANAGING STRESS

Stress comes in two varieties: good and bad. Although the two are very different, both varieties may quicken the heartbeat, raise the blood pressure, tense the muscles, and increase the flow of perspiration.

Good stress energizes us to meet the challenge of the moment. It enables a 110-pound mother to defend her child against an attacking dog, a firefighter to enter a burning building to save an elderly man, and a mountain climber to call up hidden reserves of strength to reach the summit.

Bad stress saps energy by making us respond to a situation, or stressor, with anger, crankiness, frustration, disappointment, worry, irritability, and other negative emotions. If you've ever queued up in the 10-items-or-less line at the supermarket only to discover that everybody in front of you has 50 items or more, you definitely know the meaning of bad stress. Supermarket lines are only one of the many stressors people face every day. (Other stressors include unreasonable deadlines, unreasonable workloads, an uncertain job future, traffic congestion, noisy neighbors, crime, pollution, balancing the checkbook, marital problems, and single parenthood.)

Many stressors are unique to our age. Take caregiving, for example. Thanks to medical and technological advancements, the life expectancy of the average American has increased about 30 years since the horse-and-buggy days. However, because not all elderly Americans are capable of independent living, the task of caring for them usually falls to their sons and daughters. And if the sons and daughters have their own children to raise, they end up doing triple duty—as workers, parents, and caregivers.

If you suffer from stress that's accompanied by such symptoms as headaches, palpitations, insomnia, appetite loss, and anxiety, you should see your physician. However, if you're like most of us, you simply need to get a better grip on your lifestyle, and the best place to begin is with the basics.

First, eat a nutritious diet that includes plenty of grains, vegetables, and fruit. Don't skip meals and don't "eat and run." A nutritious, well-balanced diet will sustain your health and make you less susceptible to the stressors around you. Second, exercise regularly to release tension and build endurance. If possible, join with others in an activity that makes exercise fun. Handball, tennis, volleyball, and bowling are some fun group activities. Third, get plenty of sleep. The next morning, energized and rested, your mind and body will be ready to meet any challenges the new day might bring.

Here are some additional tips that will help make your life more bearable—and enjoyable:

- Avoid nicotine and caffeine. They can jangle your nerves and make you irritable.
- Avoid resorting to alcohol to relieve tension. Alcohol is a depressant and will only make you feel worse in the long run.
- Treat yourself to an occasional relaxing massage.
- Learn to laugh at yourself and see the humorous side of life. Play practical jokes, rent or go see a funny movie, and dress up in silly costumes with your children on Halloween.
- If you have an elderly loved one to care for, don't try to do everything yourself. Instead, take advantage of community nursing services or day-care centers for the elderly. You may be eligible for financial assistance. Another option is to ask relatives to spell you

on occasion by taking the elderly person in for a week, or perhaps a weekend.

- Educate yourself about stress-reduction techniques such as meditation and deep-breathing exercises (see Using Relaxation Techniques, page 39).
- If minor annoyances—such as loud music and waiting in long lines at the supermarket—stress you, try to figure out a way around them. For example, if junior likes to listen to heavy metal music in the next room, buy him a pair of headphones for his birthday. If you want to avoid waiting in long lines at the supermarket, shop during off-hours. If you can't handle the traffic congestion, take a different, scenic route home.
- In addition to your yearly two- or three-week vacation, take occasional weekend vacations. If you have children, go on picnics, take hikes, or visit amusement parks.

Of course, there are some stressors in life—such as the IRS, inclement weather, congenital illness, and death—that are totally beyond your control. So, rather than focusing on those events you cannot change, focus instead on events you can. Begin by taping a copy of Reinhold Niebuhr's famous admonition to your refrigerator:

"God grant us grace to accept with serenity the things that cannot be changed, courage to change the things which should be changed, and the wisdom to distinguish the one from the other."

PEACEFUL LIVING

To country folk, one of the best remedies for afflictions of the spirit is the fishing pole. If you take one in hand and sneak off to a stream that nobody knows about, you'll catch a whole passel of peace and contentment, to say nothing of a trout or two.

"God never did make a more calm, quiet, innocent recreation than angling," Izaak Walton wrote more than three centuries ago. It's a fair bet that many a country doctor before and since Walton has prescribed the fishing remedy to harried patients. The hiking remedy isn't bad either. All you need to do is put on a pair of sturdy boots and head off to a patch of woods, preferably where moss carpets the earth and the smell of pine scents the air.

It's pleasurable escapes such as these—little vacations from the daily grind—that help many people prevent the molehills of distress they face every day from growing into mountains of anguish. Who, after all, can be tense when he's face to face with a chipmunk or taking an impromptu nap in the shade of tall sycamores, birches, and hemlocks?

Peace and contentment. These feelings are as precious to our minds as good health is to our bodies.

But how do you achieve peace and contentment when there are so many forces working against you in this fast-paced, survival-of-the-fittest world? What should you do if your mental pain hangs on, leechlike, in spite of your best efforts—fishing trips, hiking excursions, and a dozen and one other remedies?

THINKING POSITIVELY

Stress breeds negative thinking. Negative thinking breeds stress. It's a vicious circle. But it doesn't have to be that way. If you begin to see the good side of things—if you can laugh and enjoy life again—your positive thinking can help chase away stress and restore peace of mind.

Today doctors realize that a positive attitude can be a crucial factor in overcoming mental and physical illness of every kind, because a positive attitude helps mobilize the healing forces within the body. So if life is getting you down, don't overlook the power within you to fight back. It can be a potent weapon.

EXERCISING VIGOROUSLY

When you're under stress, the tension that builds remains inside you, much as steam remains in a tightly covered pot of boiling water. However, if you exercise, you give your body a way to release that pent-up tension and energy. If you really get your heart pumping for a good piece of time, you may be able to achieve a heightened sense of well-being. Here's why: When you

HEALTH BENEFITS

Think you're too old to begin an exercise program? Well, think again. Here are just a couple of good reasons to start working out:

- Physical activity in elders has been linked to the prevention of some cancers as well as reduced risk of heart disease, hypertension, osteoporosis, obesity, type II diabetes, and osteosclerosis.

- Adults who maintain high levels of cardiovascular endurance, strength, and flexibility are less likely to need long-term care. Increased strength, improved posture, and body control helps individuals function independently.

- Exercise puts your mind at ease. Working out helps you overcome stress, loneliness, depression, and anxiety.

exercise vigorously—for example, if you ride a bike or walk a country mile—your pituitary gland secretes feel-good hormones called endorphins that actually help to raise your spirits. Some good stress-busting activities to consider include walking, jogging, swimming, bicycling, skiing, and dancing.

MAINTAINING NUTRITION

When there's a small war going on inside you, you need a steady supply of ammunition—that is, nutritious food—to hold your own. Although your appetite may fall off, you should not skip meals or live on pork rinds. That can cause nutritional deficiencies and make you more vulnerable to all sorts of illnesses. Also, don't gorge on food to smother your stress. Doing so can result in stomach distress and perhaps an entirely new problem: weight gain.

GETTING ENOUGH REST

Sleep deprivation can aggravate the stress you're under, whatever the cause, resulting in impaired concentration, forgetfulness, and irritability. In addition, it can increase your likelihood of having an accident or developing an illness.

In other words, inadequate sleep can spell big trouble. How much sleep is the right amount? That depends on the individual. Some people need only six hours of sleep each night; they wake up alongside the early bird. Others need eight to ten hours of sleep before they can face the day. Your body will tell you whether you need more or less. If you're under a lot of stress, don't be surprised if you feel more tired than usual. During stressful times, your body may require additional hours of sleep.

USING RELAXATION TECHNIQUES

Most of us wouldn't describe a warm bath or a walk in the park as a "relaxation technique." But that's exactly what these activities are. In fact, anything that calms our spirit—smelling a rose, playing the harmonica, viewing a sunset—is a relaxation technique. The following relaxation exercises are a bit more elaborate, but research has proven them to be very effective in countering stress.

Progressive muscle relaxation. This technique alleviates tension and stress and leaves you feeling re-

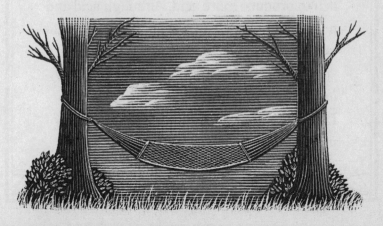

ULCER UPDATE

For almost a century, doctors believed lifestyle factors such as stress and diet caused ulcers. Today, research shows that most ulcers develop as a result of infection with bacteria called *Helicobacter pylori (H. pylori)*. According to the National Institute of Diabetes and Digestive and Kidney Diseases, the bacteria produce substances that weaken the stomach's protective mucus and make the stomach more susceptible to the damaging effects of the digestive fluids, acid and pepsin. *H. pylori* can also cause the stomach to produce more acid. Although acid and pepsin and lifestyle factors (such as physical stress, drinking alcohol or caffeine, and smoking) play a role in ulcer formation, *H. pylori* is now considered the primary cause. Doctors treat ulcers with several types of medicine, including antibiotics.

laxed and refreshed. This exercise involves consciously tensing your muscles, then relaxing them. (With repeated use of the technique, you may be able to recognize and relieve muscle tension without purposely tensing your muscles.) Here are the steps to take:

1. Lie down in a quiet place and close your eyes.
2. Tense your lips by pursing them. Hold the position for five seconds, then relax your lips.
3. Tense your forehead, facial, and neck muscles, holding the tension for five seconds each time.
4. Proceed downward, alternately tensing and relaxing different muscle groups. Continue until you have tensed and relaxed all of your muscles, including those in your toes.

Relaxation response. This widely used relaxation technique involves sitting in a chair and repeating a word. Here's what you do:

1. Sit in a comfortable chair in a quiet place and close your eyes.
2. Relax your muscles, beginning with the muscles of your feet. Progress upward, relaxing muscles as you go, until all the muscles of the body, including facial muscles, are relaxed.
3. Breathe slowly and evenly through your nose. As you breathe out, silently say a calming word or phrase of your choice (called a *mantra*) to help block out distracting or negative thoughts. Some of you may prefer saying a short prayer.

4. Continue this exercise for 10 to 20 minutes. Don't worry about how well you are performing the technique. Focus on your mantra.
5. Conclude the exercise by sitting quietly another minute or two with your eyes closed, then open your eyes and sit quietly a few minutes more.

Deep breathing. When you're under stress, you may breathe rapidly, taking in only a little air at a time. This type of breathing can promote stress. However, breathing slowly and deeply appears to counteract the stress reactions, returning your body systems to normal.

The deep breathing technique is quite simple to perform: While sitting or lying down, breathe deeply through your nose. Don't rush—feel as if you are slowly filling the pit of your stomach with air. Then slowly breathe out. Breathe deeply again, filling up your abdomen and chest. When you exhale, allow your tensions to flow out of you. Continue for two to five minutes. Repeat the exercise several times a day or whenever you feel stress building.

SEEKING COUNSEL

If you don't respond to the above self-help therapies— or if your stress is severe—your doctor may recommend that you make an appointment with a psychiatrist or other therapist. Some people resist this option. Seeing a "shrink," they believe, will stigmatize them as weak. Actually, seeking professional help is a sign of strength; it demonstrates that you are ready to attack a problem head-on.

The psychiatrist will take a medical history, evaluate your symptoms, and help you identify the cause of your distress. The psychiatrist may offer immediate short-term relief in the form of medication, although drug therapy isn't always necessary. The doctor will also help you develop a long-term solution that focuses on lifestyle adjustments.

BATTLING DEPRESSION

What if you suffer from sadness that is intense and severe—it's not simply the blues? What if your sadness is continuous and unrelenting and you feel dejected, worthless, and hopelessly alone? Then you may be suffering from clinical depression, a condition that is not to be fooled with.

Clinical depression can develop in reaction to the major stressors that will afflict many of us at some point in our lives: the death of a spouse, the death of a close relative, divorce, separation, financial loss, loss of employment, retirement, health problems, sexual problems, and lifestyle changes. In addition, clinical depression can occur as a result of chemical imbalances in the

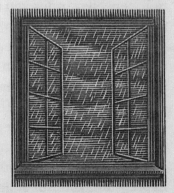

body. Scientists now believe that genetic factors may also make certain individuals more susceptible to experiencing episodes of depression.

In addition to extreme sadness, victims of depression may develop the following symptoms: loss of interest in life, diminished or increased appetite, insomnia or excessive sleeping, fatigue, constipation, chest pain, achiness, indecision, feelings of guilt over minor matters, and episodes of crying.

If you believe you may be suffering from clinical depression, your first priority should be to see your physician. Because some of the symptoms of depression mimic those of physical illnesses, the doctor will conduct an examination and take a medical history. If the results rule out underlying physical illnesses and confirm that you have depression, the physician will probably recommend an antidepressant medication that will begin to alleviate your symptoms in two to six weeks. The physician will either prescribe the medication himself or refer you to a psychiatrist who specializes in treating depression. In addition to drug therapy, your doctor may also recommend cognitive therapy, psychotherapy, or group therapy to help you gain insight into your problems and develop long-term coping skills to deal with difficult times.

As your depression begins to lift, don't assume that the medication will purge you of all daily tension and stress. Like the person you were before you developed depression, you will still react negatively on occasion to stressors such as financial problems and work dead-lines—everyone does. But to keep depression at bay, do your best to stay in tip-top mental and physical condition. Eat right. Exercise. Get enough sleep. Avoid tobacco and alcohol. And regularly practice relaxation techniques.

MANAGING ANXIETY

Anxiety is a form of stress. Generally, it refers to the uneasy feeling you experience when confronted with a threat to your mental or physical well-being.

For example, you might become anxious about giving a speech. You wonder, *What if I appear nervous and confused, or suffer a memory lapse?* Or, you might fret over a recurring pain in your abdomen. *What if I have to have an operation? What if it's cancer?* As you mull the possibilities, your hands perspire, your heartbeat quickens, and butterflies play tag in your stomach.

Everyone who is human suffers this kind of anxiety from time to time. As long as episodes of anxiety are infrequent and of short duration, they should not concern you. However, if anxiety begins to rule your emotions, frequently making you nervous and queasy over everyday tasks and responsibilities—or over vague, unexplained fears—you increase your risk of developing serious health problems.

In less severe cases, victims of anxiety may experience rapid breathing, rapid heartbeat, muscle tension, muscle twitching, insomnia, fatigue, sweaty palms, and lack of appetite. In severe cases, victims may suffer from panic attacks. During these attacks, victims experience some or all of these symptoms: racing heartbeat, chest pain, dizziness, difficulty breathing, profuse sweating, nausea, trembling, choking, numbness, and fear of dying.

Many people who suffer a panic attack never have another. Others may have frequent attacks. In the latter case, the victim may begin to worry incessantly about when the next attack will occur, and this anxiety breeds even more anxiety. In extreme cases, the victim may avoid going to the mall, to the supermarket, or even to work for fear of suffering an anxiety attack.

If you are suffering from any form of anxiety that interferes with normal living, see your physician. The doctor will probably conduct a physical exam and order laboratory tests to check for an underlying illness that could be causing the anxiety. (Some ailments, such as an overactive thyroid gland, can produce anxiety symptoms.) If your physician rules out a physical cause, he may recommend treatment options such as drug therapy and self-help strategies.

COPING WITH GRIEF

Grief is a part of life. You cannot avoid it and you should not try to. Instead, confront it, and let it run its course. Along the way, do not suppress your feelings. Doing so will only postpone or prolong your grief while intensifying your bottled-up stress.

Initially you may react to the loss of a loved one with shock, disbelief, and profound sadness. Later, you may feel lonely, helpless, and confused. You may even feel anger, wanting to blame someone for the loss—even yourself. Because you are under stress, you may develop palpitations, shortness of breath, insomnia, and other symptoms. Realize, though, that experiencing such symptoms is to be expected during these tough times.

Both men and women should not be afraid to cry. After all, your tears are paying tribute to the life of the loved one; they are a form of eulogy. And tears provide an outlet for your emotional stress.

Don't be afraid to talk about your feelings. Airing them will help you make sense of the loss and speed your acceptance of it. It will also help you deal with any sense of guilt you may be feeling over some past hurt you may have caused the deceased. Women, it has been said, tend to cope better than men in times of loss because they are quick to seek out the company of a sympathetic listener. If you are a man, take a lesson from the women around you.

Understanding grief and learning how to cope with its varied emotions can be very difficult. If you believe you need the guidance of a physician or therapist to help you through your grief, don't hesitate to contact one. The loss of a loved one is, after all, a major trauma. (Seeking the help of a professional may also be advisable if you are currently trying to cope with other distress, such as a serious health condition or an upsetting lifestyle change.)

Because grieving is a sad time, many mourners seek quick fixes or magic bullets to make them feel good again. Alcohol and feverish activities such as wild shopping sprees are among those strategies that really don't eliminate grief; they merely cover up the variety of emotions you may be experiencing. When the alcohol high evaporates or the shine wears off the new shoes, the grief will reappear, waiting to be confronted.

Bear in mind, however, that grieving doesn't mean that you'll feel gloomy all the time. There is nothing improper or unhealthy about laughing or enjoying leisure activities during a grieving period. Nor is there anything wrong with recalling humorous incidents involving the deceased loved one. In fact, it's simply good therapy to do so.

Following are additional suggestions to help you through a time of loss:

- Don't neglect your diet. Early on, be sure to drink plenty of liquids to replenish fluid lost through heightened nervous activity.
- Continue your exercise routine. Exercise will help relieve tension and make you tired enough to sleep.
- If you have a mind to, visit the grave of the loved one whenever and as often as you like.
- If you are now alone, consider getting a pet to keep you company. Research shows that a dog or cat can do wonders for sagging spirits.

- Avoid dwelling on what you didn't do for the deceased person. Instead, take comfort in those things you did do.

A FINAL WORD...

Stress, depression, and grief will invade all our lives at some time or another. Most of the time, the symptoms will be minor and relatively easy to manage. Relief can come swiftly if we reach out for help. Asking for help is a "technique" that isn't often discussed, but it is one that is just as important as other types of treatment. We all need to learn to ask for help; none of us is so self-sufficient as to have all the answers.

HEALING WAYS

In this chapter, you're likely to stumble across a variety of remedies for practically everything that ails you—from backaches and headaches to insomnia and sunburn. Some recommendations may seem familiar, and some may not. Why not give them a try? Sometimes a simple homespun remedy is all it takes to get you back on your feet again.

ALLERGIES

Blame it on your immune system. Its purpose is to preserve your well-being by attacking invading germs. But sometimes it gets a little paranoid and attacks harmless foods, drugs, and aromas, as well as materials that have the audacity to come in contact with your skin.

You can be allergic to almost anything—a food, drug, fabric, chemical, metal, cosmetic, aroma, plant, or even the ink on a printed page. Some folks are even allergic to certain soaps and deodorants, which, in turn, can make people "allergic" to them.

When the immune system targets a threat, it releases its most powerful warriors—antibodies. When the antibodies attack, the body releases excessive amounts of certain chemicals, including histamines. The result? A variety of allergy-related symptoms.

CAUSES

Allergy triggers include milk, shellfish, wheat, eggs, soybeans, and nuts; windborne pollens from ragweed, sagebrush, Russian thistle, and other plants; windborne pollens from trees and grasses; poison ivy, poison oak, and poison sumac; detergents, soaps, and cosmetics; metal; wool and feathers; adhesive tape; dust and dust mites; smoke and chemical vapors; animal fur or dander (dry skin); mold; and insect stings and bites.

SYMPTOMS

Allergy symptoms may include runny nose, watery eyes, swollen sinuses, swollen mouth or throat, sneezing, rash, itching, hives, nausea, vomiting, diarrhea, and abdominal pain.

REMEDIES

- Identify the cause of your allergy. Then remove it or avoid it. If you haven't a clue to the cause, keep a diary. Record your daily activities—where you go, what you eat, and so on. Record the date and time when you experience allergy symptoms. In time, you'll discover what's provoking your symptoms.
- If pollen is your problem, avoid close encounters with pollen-producing vegetation when you're out-

doors. When indoors, run an air cleaner or an air conditioner to filter out the offenders.

- Dehumidify your dust mites. These almost invisible creatures—which inhabit carpets, clothing, curtains, and anything else that gathers dust—absolutely abhor dry air. Take away their moisture and you'll take away their mischief.
- When cleaning your house, don't raise dust with dry cloths and feather dusters. Instead, use dampened mops, cloths, and sponges to wipe up the dust.
- Replace furnace filters often. Doing so will rid you of a prime source of pollen and dust buildup.
- Wash clothing and bedding often to remove potential allergens.
- If you work around vapors known to cause allergic reactions, wear a protective mask.
- Take an over-the-counter antihistamine to relieve such symptoms as runny nose, watery eyes, and sneezing.
- Ban smoking in your home. Cigarette, cigar, and pipe smoke are common causes of allergic reactions.
- If an allergy-causing pet is too precious to part with, make sure your little friend gets regular baths and haircuts to remove pollen, dust mites, and other allergens the animal may be harboring.

Call your physician if you are unable to identify the cause of your allergy. The doctor can conduct tests that may pinpoint the cause.

ARTHRITIS

Edward Schneider, a scientist at the National Institute on Aging, tells the following story: A 95-year-old arthritis patient walked into his doctor's office and complained about pain in his right knee. The doctor told him he had to expect pain in his knee after 95 years.

"But," the man said, "my left knee is 95 years old, too, and it's doing just fine."

Arthritis, like other diseases, can be unpredictable and sometimes downright fickle. Not only is arthritis bothersome to knee joints, but it also can affect other joints in the body, causing pain, swelling, and stiffness.

There are more than 100 varieties of arthritis, afflicting nearly 40 million Americans. The two most common varieties are osteoarthritis and rheumatoid arthritis.

With osteoarthritis, there is a wearing away of cartilage in the joints. Healthy cartilage is the elastic tissue that lines and cushions the joints and allows bones to move smoothly against one another. When this cartilage deteriorates, the bones rub together, causing pain and swelling. Osteoarthritis can cause permanent damage and deformity of the joints. The disease generally develops after age 45, most often targeting the joints of the knees, hips, fingers, spine, and neck. Doctors and patients sometimes refer to osteoarthritis as "wear and tear" arthritis.

Rheumatoid arthritis can attack at any age. This form of arthritis affects the connective tissues as well as the body's organs. In rheumatoid arthritis, the synovium (the thin membrane that lines and lubricates the joints) becomes inflamed. The inflammation eventually destroys the cartilage. As scar tissue gradually replaces the damaged cartilage, the joints become misshaped and rigid. Rheumatoid arthritis may also damage the heart, lungs, nerves, and eyes.

Diagnosis of arthritis requires a physical examination. X-ray studies and laboratory tests may also be recommended for confirmation of joint swelling and to determine the extent of tissue damage. With appropriate treatment, however, most folks who have arthritis can lead normal—and active—lives.

CAUSES

Osteoarthritis: Causes of osteoarthritis include gradual wear and tear of a joint, injury to a joint, and complications of other illnesses, such as diabetes. According to Lawrence M. Tierney, Jr., M.D., professor of medicine at the University of California at San Francisco, osteoarthritis is so common that 90 percent of all Americans develop some signs of the disease in the weight-bearing joints (such as knees and hips) by age 40.

Rheumatoid arthritis: The precise cause of rheumatoid arthritis is unknown. Some researchers believe that a virus may trigger the disease, causing an autoimmune response whereby the body attacks its own tissues.

SYMPTOMS

Osteoarthritis: Symptoms of osteoarthritis include joint pain, stiffness, limited mobility, and sometimes, upon movement, cracking sounds. Usually there is no inflammation or redness. If the disease afflicts the spine, you may have pain in the neck and lower back. If osteoarthritis afflicts the hips and knees, you may walk with a limp. The symptoms may come and go, allowing pain-free intervals that last for months, sometimes even years. The intensity of symptoms can range from very mild to very severe.

Rheumatoid arthritis: Symptoms of rheumatoid arthritis include joint pain, redness, and stiffness that occur upon waking. Bony nodules may appear under the skin.

REMEDIES

The goals of arthritis therapy are to relieve pain and inflammation, maintain or improve mobility, and prevent further deterioration. The following remedies are designed to help achieve these goals.

• Go swimming. Swimming helps maintain joint function and flexibility without stressing the joints. Moreover, it gets you into the company of others.

- Stretch. Stretching exercises keep joints in good working condition, maintain flexibility, and help relieve stiffness. For information on safe stretching exercises, check with your local chapter of the Arthritis Foundation.
- Ride a bike. Bike riding is also a form of exercise that won't jar your joints. Use caution and ride on smooth surfaces in off-street locales. Wear protective clothing, knee pads, and a helmet.
- Take a simple walk in the woods. Pick berries. Forage for herbs. Walking is linked to a host of health benefits, including fighting coronary heart disease, aiding in the treatment of high blood pressure, and battling depression.
- Maintain your ideal weight. Being overweight can worsen arthritic conditions because excess weight can stress weight-bearing joints.
- Balance activity and rest. Being overactive can unduly stress your joints, but underactivity can turn them into rusty gates. Rest when your body tells you to and exercise when the spirit calls.
- Protect your joints. Don't lift, reach, or bend beyond your ability. Use a ladder when picking apples or sit on a stool when picking strawberries. If your fingers pain you, use the palm of your hand to screw the cap on the mayonnaise jar. Marian Minor, Ph.D., assistant professor of physical therapy at the University of Missouri at Columbia, offers these additional tips to help protect arthritic hands:

WORK IT OUT

D id you know that exercise is one of the most important steps you can take to help relieve the pain of arthritis? Exercise increases the strength and flexibility of the muscles and ligaments surrounding the joints. It also helps maintain and increase the strength of bones. Falls, the major cause of fatal injuries in people over 75 years of age, can be reduced dramatically through participation in exercises that improve balance and mobility.

In order to get the greatest benefit from your exercise regimen, you should try to get a workout in every day. And because exercising in water reduces the weight on joints, swimming or other water exercises (including water aerobics) is ideal for most people with arthritis.

- —Use both hands to pick up a coffee mug instead of curling fingers around the handle.
- —Use your hips to close kitchen drawers.
- —Hang a strap from the handle of a cupboard or refrigerator door. To open doors, place your forearm through the strap loop and pull.

- Dig out that hot water bottle. Heat treatments can relieve chronic joint pain and muscle stiffness. (You also can try taking a hot shower or using a heating pad or an electric blanket.) Do not apply heat for more than 20 minutes at a time.

- Apply cold. Cold treatments are best for acute inflammation, swelling, and muscle spasms. (A frozen bag of peas makes a great ice pack.) Do not apply cold for more than 20 minutes at a time.

- Apply heat and cold. Some people gain relief by first soaking a joint in warm water, then cold water, then warm water, etc., for up to 20 minutes at a time.

- Use relaxation techniques. When you're tense or anxious, your muscles tighten, increasing arthritis pain. Relaxation techniques (see page 39) can help alleviate daily tensions and anxiety.

- Choose the right painkiller. Which should you use? If you have osteoarthritis but no inflammation, try acetaminophen. If you have inflammation and pain from rheumatoid arthritis, try aspirin or another nonsteroidal anti-inflammatory drug (NSAIDs) such as ibuprofen. If you're prone to stomach upset, try using coated tablets; they may reduce the risk of stomach

COVER YOUR BACK

There's no better time to watch your back than when you travel. Follow these simple tips to avoid back pain:

- Use luggage with wheels whenever possible, even if you aren't walking very far.
- Ask for help when placing bags in overhead compartments.
- Bend slowly and carefully when storing your belongings under the seat in front of you. Ask someone for help if the items are too heavy.
- Be careful when retrieving your bags. Remember, when you pull, you are using the muscles in your lower back.
- When sitting, give your muscles a break by changing your position occasionally.
- Dress in loose, comfortable clothing so you can easily stretch cramped, aching muscles.

irritation. Be aware that pain relievers can cause adverse side effects. Long-term use of acetaminophen can cause liver or kidney damage. Painkillers can interact with other drugs; if you are currently taking other medications, check with your physician before attempting to treat arthritis with over-the-counter remedies. A pregnant woman should not take a medication without her doctor's approval.

- Be upbeat. Negative emotions, such as worry and frustration, can increase your perception of pain.

Call your physician if remedies bring no relief, your symptoms seem to worsen, or you have unexplained symptoms.

BACK PAIN

You heave the saddle up on the horse and—ouch!—there goes your back. It's out again.

Eight of every ten Americans suffer episodes of back pain sometime in their lives. The pain may be mild or moderate, or it may be excruciating, making it difficult to perform even simple everyday tasks like tying your shoes. Strains, the most common cause of back pain, occur when overworked or under-exercised back muscles are pushed beyond their limits.

CAUSES

Many people experience back pain as they age and their joint tissues deteriorate or shift. Back pain can also be caused by sitting for long periods of time; psychological tension; diseases of the kidneys, heart, lungs, intestinal tract, or reproductive organs; osteoporosis; physical malformations; and being overweight. A slipped disk, muscle sprain, ligament strain, sudden twisting or turning motion, kidney infection, bone disease, tumor, pregnancy, and menstrual cramps can also cause back pain.

SYMPTOMS

Backaches can occur abruptly after physical activity or may develop slowly. The pain may feel like a sharp jab or a dull ache. Severe back pain may also be accompanied by pain or numbness radiating down one or both legs. Most muscular back pain disappears in a week or two, whereas some aches and pains can last up to two months or more.

REMEDIES

- To help keep inflammation and discomfort to a minimum, apply ice to the strained area within 24 hours of the injury. (A bag of frozen peas makes a great ice pack!) Don't put the ice pack directly on your skin, however. To avoid cold injury to the tissues, wrap the bag in a thin towel and place it on the injured area for 20 minutes. Take a 30 minute break, then apply the ice pack again for 20 minutes more.

- If it's been more than 24 hours since you injured your back, apply heat to help relieve muscle spasms, because ice will no longer reduce pain or inflammation. A 20-minute soak in the bathtub may be all it takes to get you on your feet again.
- Exercise as soon as you're able. But don't pitch hay or dig a potato field. And don't lift heavy objects or engage in other activities that may unduly stress the back.
- Sit straight to relieve pressure on your spine and back muscles. If you work at a desk, sit close to it and use a foot rest to elevate your knees just above your hips.
- When sitting, shift position from time to time. Every 30 minutes or so, stand up and walk around or try a stretching exercise. The American Academy of Orthopaedic Surgeons recommends the following exercise for preventing back pain: With your feet several inches apart, place your hands on your lower back and slowly bend backward while keeping your knees straight. Bend back as far as you can and hold your position for a few seconds. Repeat.
- Sleep on your side on a supportive mattress. Sleeping on your stomach stresses your lower back. When getting out of bed, take it easy. Remember to roll or slide out of bed, rather than quickly "jerking" yourself up.

- Lose weight. Extra weight puts extra strain on back muscles. Sensible, gradual weight loss can help ease back pain.
- Store heavy objects above waist level so you can lift them without stressing your back.
- When lifting an object off the floor, bend your knees without bending your waist. Look straight ahead and keep your shoulders up. If an object feels too heavy, don't try to lift it yourself.

Call your physician if symptoms such as fever, nausea, vomiting, chest pain, dizziness, rapid weight loss, abdominal pain, or sudden bowel or bladder incontinence accompany your back pain; if back pain radiates down your leg; or if you experience prolonged back pain (lasting for more than one or two weeks).

BITES AND STINGS

No matter where you live, you're at risk of being stung by an insect or bitten by an animal. And bites and stings can be dangerous if the insect is a disease-carrier or the biting animal is poisonous or has rabies.

In some instances, the sting of a bee, hornet, yellow jacket, spider, or other insect can cause some individuals to suffer anaphylactic shock. Symptoms of this life-threatening allergic reaction usually occur within minutes of the sting and include tingling or numbness, breathing difficulty, rapid pulse, a rapid decrease in

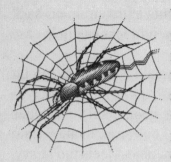

blood pressure, hives, tightness in the chest, and faintness. Emergency medical treatment usually consists of an epinephrine injection. In some cases, a corticosteroid may be given as well to lessen existing symptoms and halt progression of the allergic reaction.

SYMPTOMS

The symptoms of bites and stings vary. Some common symptoms include pain, burning, itching, redness, inflammation, welts, and hives.

REMEDIES

To treat bee stings:
- Remove the stinger immediately.
- Run cold water over the sting area—or apply an ice pack—to relieve the burning sensation and minimize swelling. Continue applying cold for 20 minutes at a time for about an hour.
- Use calamine lotion or the oral antihistamine Benadryl to alleviate itching and swelling in the area.

To treat mosquito, fly, and spider bites:
- Wash the bite thoroughly with soap and water.
- Apply an ice pack to the affected area for about 15 minutes to reduce pain, inflammation, and itching.

- Try taking an over-the-counter antihistamine to further quell the itch. Don't use this remedy, though, if you're pregnant.
- Persons with known sensitivity to insect bites should carry kits with injectable epinephrine.

To treat tick bites:
Don't assume the tiny tick is a harmless creature. Some ticks carry Lyme disease and Rocky Mountain spotted fever, which can lead to serious complications. If you're bitten by a tick, here's what to do:
- To remove a tick, grasp the insect with tweezers and slowly pull straight upward. Use the tweezers to remove any remaining parts of the tick. Save the tick in a small jar of alcohol, so that if a suspicious infection develops, the tick can be analyzed for disease.
- Do not use a lighted match to try to remove the insect. This method doesn't work and can cause serious burns.
- Thoroughly wash the bite area and your hands with soap and water.
- Apply alcohol or hydrogen peroxide to the bite, then cover it with a bandage.
- There is no need to see a doctor unless you notice any signs of swelling or redness around the bite (a sign of infection); a bull's-eye-shaped rash (often a symptom of Lyme disease); or fever, chills, muscle aches, nausea, or skin rash. (Symptoms may not develop until several weeks after the bite occurred.)

To treat animal bites:

If you are bitten by an animal that's not familiar to you, assume that it's rabid. Wash the wound for 10 or 15 minutes to remove the saliva, and call your physician. If possible, ask the local animal shelter to catch the animal for analysis; if the animal is rabid, you will need rabies shots.

To treat non-rabid bites, follow this advice:

- Thoroughly wash the bite area with soap and water. It may take four or five minutes to remove all the saliva.
- Apply an antibiotic cream to fight infection.
- If there is very minor bleeding, cover the wound with sterile gauze.
- Watch for fever, skin redness, or increasing pain.
- Call your physician if an animal bite (including human bites) has broken the skin. You may be due for a tetanus shot.
- If there is major bleeding or a puncture wound, apply pressure to the wound with your hand, making sure not to cut off circulation, says Michael O. Fleming, M.D., a family practitioner at Highland Hospital in Shreveport, Louisiana. (You can also try loosely tying a cloth around the wound.) See your physician or go to a hospital emergency room.

To treat snakebites:

If a snake has bitten you, you are not necessarily in imminent danger. (For one thing, the snake may not be poisonous. If it is poisonous, its bite may not have broken your skin. If its bite did break the skin, it may not have injected its poison.) Lie down and remain calm. Do not eat or drink anything, especially alcoholic beverages. If possible, have a companion perform the following tasks:

- Elevate the limb and apply a cold compress. Do not use ice. Doing so may worsen tissue damage.
- Tie a loose tourniquet or tight band two to four inches above the bite. Do not cut off blood flow; make sure you can feel a pulse below the tourniquet. If swelling occurs at the site of the tourniquet, move it several inches higher.
- Arrange transportation to the nearest hospital.
- Identify the snake, if possible. Your knowledge will help emergency physicians determine the type of venom that may have been injected.

Call your physician if you react to drugs used to treat the bite or you require additional supportive treatment such as wound cleaning.

BURNS

You're pan-frying freshly caught trout when suddenly hot grease splatters onto the back of your hand. Neighbors two pastures over can hear you shout.

How serious is the burn? Can you treat it at home or should you go to the hospital?

A first-degree burn usually is not too serious because it damages only the outer layer of the skin, or epidermis. You can treat it yourself if the burn does not affect a large area of your body.

A second-degree burn involves the epidermis and the layer of skin below it, called the dermis. You can usually treat a second-degree burn at home if the burn is no more than two inches across and no infection develops.

A third-degree burn affects all layers of skin and destroys nerves. Always receive emergency treatment for this type of burn.

CAUSES

Causes of burns include fire, steam, sunlight, radiation, chemicals, high temperatures, and electricity.

SYMPTOMS

First-degree burn: Symptoms of first-degree burn include redness, tenderness, and swelling, but no blistering of the skin.

Second-degree burn: Symptoms include redness, tenderness, swelling, blistering, and possibly infection of the skin.

Third-degree burn: Skin may appear black or white. Because third-degree burns often destroy nerves, initially, victims may feel no pain.

REMEDIES

- Immediately douse the burn area with a clean, cold liquid, such as milk, juice, or water. The coolness will actually stop the burn from spreading.
- Run cool tap water over the burn for up to 15 minutes.
- Do not wash the burn with soap and water. Do not apply an antibiotic spray or cream to prevent infection. Do not apply butter, margarine, or petroleum jelly. (If you have a blistering second-degree burn, these agents can lead to infection.)
- If you cannot run tap water over the burn because of its location, apply a cool, wet compress. Do not apply an ice cube directly to the skin because frostbite might occur.
- Avoid touching the burned area. Do not break or pick at blisters. Doing so will increase the risk of infection.
- Protect the burn by covering it with a sterile dressing. Change the dressing daily.
- Take aspirin or ibuprofen to reduce pain or inflammation.
- Expect up to three weeks for the burn to heal.

Call your physician if the burn forms a scab immediately; you have a blistering burn larger than two inches across; you have a first-degree burn that covers a large area of your body; the skin around the burn area feels numb; the burn does not appear to be healing; there is spreading redness near the burn; or you develop a fever. If an infant has suffered any kind of burn, call your doctor.

COLDS

Medical researchers have yet to discover a cure for the common cold. It's no wonder: Any of hundreds of viruses can cause the contagious upper-respiratory infection. Colds generally involve the membranes of the voice box, throat, and nose, but they also can involve the breathing tubes (the trachea and its two branches, called bronchi) leading to the lungs.

CAUSES

Although colds are caused by viruses, factors such as stress, anxiety, fatigue, smoking, and nutritional problems can all increase your risk of developing a cold.

SYMPTOMS

Symptoms include coughing, sneezing, hoarseness, nasal and sinus congestion, mild fever, sore throat, fatigue, watery eyes, and loss of appetite.

REMEDIES

- Throw a few extra logs on the fireplace, relax, and get plenty of bed rest.
- Take aspirin or acetaminophen to help relieve body aches and headache. Children and teenagers should not be given aspirin for a viral infection because of

the risk of Reye syndrome, a rare but serious illness reported to be associated with aspirin.

- Take an antihistamine to relieve congestion. Be aware, though, that antihistamines can cause drowsiness. And while decongestants also relieve nasal congestion, they can make you feel jittery and cause insomnia. Some folks prefer taking a decongestant during the day and an antihistamine at night.
- Drink plenty of fluids to help thin lung secretions and prevent dehydration. Avoid milk, though; in some people, it may thicken lung secretions.
- Help yourself to a hearty bowl of chicken soup—a traditional remedy that really works. Because it's liquid, it helps prevent dehydration and thins mucus secretions. Because it's hot, it may help promote blood circulation in your throat, speeding healing. Because it contains salt, it may reduce throat swelling. Also, its steamy vapors may help relieve nasal congestion.
- Use a cool-mist vaporizer or climb into a hot shower to further thin mucus secretions.
- Apply petroleum jelly to the outside of your nostrils to relieve rawness caused by frequent nose blowing.
- Vitamin C may reduce the severity of your symptoms or the duration of your cold. Stick to a dosage of no more than 2,000 milligrams a day. Higher doses of vitamin C may cause diarrhea.

Call your physician if you develop white or yellow spots on your throat; you are short of breath; you have a fever that occurs five days after your cold begins; you cough up yellow-green or grayish sputum; you experience pain in the chest area, ears, or sinuses; or you are unusually lethargic.

CONSTIPATION

For some, regularity means having a bowel movement three times a week; for others, it is part of their daily routine. What matters is not the frequency of your bowel movements, but whether your normal routine alters. Sudden changes in bowel habits may be a sign of a serious underlying illness.

CAUSES

Constipation is most commonly caused by a lack of dietary fiber. But stress, failure to drink enough liquids, depression, overuse of laxatives, and adverse reactions to drugs may also be responsible. Possible underlying causes of constipation are kidney disease, cancer, an underactive thyroid gland, tearing of anal tissue, and excessive calcium in the blood.

SYMPTOMS

Symptoms of constipation include fewer-than-usual bowel movements, straining, hard stools, and sometimes pain and bleeding in the rectal area.

REMEDIES

- Begin each day with a high-fiber cereal. Cereals containing 5 grams of fiber or more per serving are best. (Check the side of the cereal box for a complete listing of its contents.)
- Drink at least eight glasses of water a day.
- Eat plenty of fruits, vegetables, and whole-grain products, which are rich in the fiber you need to promote bowel movements.
- Try natural laxatives such as prunes, dates, and figs. A commercial product that contains psyllium may also be helpful.
- Allow enough time in your daily schedule for nature to take its course. Go when you feel the urge.
- Exercise vigorously. It'll help speed digested food through the bowels. Walk. Play tennis. Go for a quick jog.
- Take time to relax. Tension and stress tend to inhibit the bowels from doing their work.
- Keep track of what you eat. If constipation regularly occurs after eating a certain food, try reducing or eliminating that food from your diet.

Call your physician if your constipation persists for more than five days, you are unable to pass gas, you bleed during a bowel movement, or you have abdominal cramps or fever.

CORNS AND CALLUSES

Into everybody's life a little corn must grow—usually, where it hurts most, on the joint of your toe.

Corns are raised bumps of thickened skin with a hard center. They form on feet as a result of constant pressure or friction. Corns are cousins of calluses, another form of thickened skin. Calluses generally develop where there is pressure or friction as well, usually on the heels or balls of the foot.

Calluses remain flush to the skin, like a carpet to a floor or a poster to a telephone poll. Calluses sometimes develop a hard center, however, and turn into corns themselves.

There are hard corns and soft corns. The hard ones usually form on toe joints or the outer side of the little toe. Soft corns prefer to form between toes.

CAUSES

Both calluses and corns are caused by rubbing, pinching, or squeezing of the skin. The skin acts as the body's protector against outside elements. Corns and calluses form when the body tries to protect an area from pressure by building up a mass of dead skin cells.

SYMPTOMS

Callus: A callus is a painless thickening of the skin.

Corn: Symptoms include pain, tenderness, and thickened skin that forms into a bump with a hard center.

REMEDIES

- Soften the corn or callus by soaking the area in warm water.
- Gently abrade the surface with a pumice stone. Apply a moisturizing cream. Repeat as often as necessary, but be careful not to irritate the skin.
- Insert cotton between the toes to inhibit the formation of soft corns.
- Do unto your feet as you would do unto other parts of your body. In other words, make your feet comfortable and buy shoes that fit well. Both corns and calluses are commonly caused by tight, ill-fitting shoes.
- Never attempt to cut away corns or calluses with a sharp instrument. Doing so could lead to a serious infection.

Call your physician if the development of corns or calluses persists despite treatment, a corn or callus becomes infected, or you require treatment for a deformity that may be causing the corns and calluses. (People who have abnormal bone structure in their feet or certain types of arthritis tend to develop corns.)

COUGHING

Coughing is a symptom, not an illness. The cough is a protective reflex: It clears your breathing passages of secretions or irritants such as smoke and dust. As long as it accomplishes this task effectively, coughing should be regarded as a normal and even healthy reaction.

A harsh or forceful cough can be an irritant to the lining of the airways, however. The act of coughing causes the airways to contract. When this happens over and over, it leads to inflamed membranes and helps to perpetuate the cough. Thus, while taking action to relieve your cough, don't ignore its root cause—especially if the cough lasts two weeks or more, if it produces bloody or greenish phlegm, or if it produces no phlegm at all.

CAUSES

Coughing can be caused by colds, flu, bronchitis, pneumonia, emphysema, lung cancer, heart disease, croup, asthma, allergies, postnasal drip, drug reactions, and irritants such as dust, tobacco smoke, and chemical fumes.

SYMPTOMS

Types of coughs include dry coughing that produces little or no phlegm (usually typical of flu and colds), wet coughing that produces phlegm (usually typical of lung infections such as bronchitis and possibly pneumonia), coughing with wheezing (a possible symptom of emphysema), and a barking cough (usually typical of croup, an infection of the vocal cords that occurs in children under age six).

Symptoms of a cough include throat soreness, chest pain or burning, a feeling of pressure in the chest, and a tickle in the throat.

REMEDIES

- If an irritant such as smoke or a chemical is causing your cough, avoid it.
- If an infection such as a cold or the flu is causing your cough, use the home remedies listed in this chapter to help alleviate your symptoms.
- Drink plenty of fluids to help thin lung secretions and prevent dehydration. Avoid milk, though; in some people, it may thicken lung secretions.
- If your cough is wet, drink fluids to soothe your throat and loosen mucus. You also may wish to try a cool-mist vaporizer as well as an over-the-counter cough medication called an expectorant.
- If your cough is dry, drink fluids, especially warm or hot ones, to soothe your throat. You may also wish to try over-the-counter cough drops that contain the drug dextromethorphan.

Call your physician if you cough up greenish or bloody phlegm, you cough up bright red blood, your cough persists even after your cold or flu disappears, or you experience chest or throat pain or breathing difficulty.

DRY EYES

Tears lubricate the eyes, protecting them against wind and dust and ridding them of bacteria. However, when your tear supply dwindles, constant blinking—as well as wind and other outside forces—can make your eyes scratchy and red. This condition is known as dry eye.

Certain medications and dry climates can irritate the eyes. Dry eye can also be caused by a disorder called Sjögren syndrome. This inflammatory disorder causes joint pain and reduces the secretions of the sweat glands, the salivary glands, and the lacrimal (tear) glands. Nine of every ten victims of Sjögren syndrome are women; the average age of onset is 50 years.

CAUSES

Possible causes of dry eye include Sjögren syndrome; medications such as oral contraceptives, antihistamines, antidepressants, antibiotics, and diuretics; dry climate; dry working or living environment; menopause; and Bell Palsy, in which individuals may have difficulty blinking.

SYMPTOMS

Symptoms of dry eye include burning and irritation, blurred vision, dry mouth, and the feeling that a foreign object is lodged in your eye. When dryness occurs in one eye only, the other eye may water excessively.

REMEDIES

- Lubricate your eyes with artificial tears, which are available over the counter at your local pharmacy. Do not confuse artificial-tears products with products designed to whiten red eyes or with eye washes designed to irrigate eyes.
- Humidify your home or office.
- If a certain medication seems to be responsible for causing dry eyes, ask your doctor whether a suitable alternative is available.
- Try to blink more often in windy conditions and when you are watching television, reading a book, or staring at a computer screen.

Call your physician if you have symptoms of Sjögren syndrome (dryness of the mucous membranes) or if dryness of the eye persists despite remedies. Failure to correct the problem can lead to tissue damage and impaired vision.

DRY MOUTH

Dry mouth is a condition in which not enough saliva is produced in the mouth. Breathing too much through your mouth—and not enough through your nose—can cause this condition. If your mouth is dry all the time, don't put off remedying the problem. Here's why: Saliva contains an antibacterial agent. When your mouth doesn't get enough of it, the process of tooth decay can increase dramatically. Also, because saliva lubricates the mouth and moistens the food you eat, it makes swallowing easier. Dry mouth can lead to tongue and lip fissures and impair your sense of taste and smell.

CAUSES

Dry mouth may be caused by Sjögren syndrome, diabetes, dehydration, diet pills, certain medications, and breathing through the mouth.

SYMPTOMS

Symptoms of dry mouth (and sometimes dry throat) include difficulty chewing or swallowing, decreased ability to taste and smell, and tongue and lip fissures.

REMEDIES

- If you have diabetes, drink plenty of water to replace the fluids lost through frequent urination.
- Increase your fluid intake if you are dehydrated as a result of activity or illness.
- If a certain medication seems to be leaving your mouth dry, ask your doctor whether a suitable alternative is available.
- If a diet pill seems to be causing the problem, discontinue using it. Instead, try exercising and eating a nutritious, low-calorie diet.

- If a stuffy nose caused by a cold is forcing you to breathe through your mouth, take a hot shower. The steam can help relieve nasal congestion (see Colds, page 70).
- Eat "chewy" meals and snacks to stimulate saliva production. Grandma's homemade granola bars might be just the ticket to give your mouth the workout it needs. Between meals, keep your mouth moving with sugar-free gum or a piece of hard candy.

Call your physician if you have symptoms of Sjögren syndrome (dryness of the mucous membranes) or diabetes or you suspect your symptoms are caused by medication you are taking.

DRY SKIN

Covering you from the top of your head to the soles of your feet, skin is a blanket of cells and nerve tissue that defends against germs, pollutants, heat, cold, ultraviolet sun rays—and a thousand and one other would-be invaders.

But while it protects your insides, your skin itself can take a beating. One of its arch enemies is dry air. When humidity falls, the air steals moisture from your skin, leaving it feeling itchy and flaky. Sometimes the skin cracks, as with chapped lips or dry knuckles.

Winter weather can be particularly hard on skin because humidity usually falls with the temperature.

Indoors, the air may be just as dry—or drier—because furnaces and fireplaces are going full blast.

But hot summer weather can hurt your skin, too, if you're among those who spend a lot of time out-of-doors. The sun's rays can bake the moisture right out of your skin, leaving it feeling rough and raw.

Cosmetics, too, can take their toll on the skin, triggering allergic reactions that have symptoms similar to those of dry skin. Finally, be aware that as you age, you're more prone to developing dry skin because the glands that moisturize your skin become less active.

CAUSES

Causes of dry skin include dry air (indoors and out), prolonged exposure to sunlight, cosmetics, aging, and excessive washing or scrubbing that removes natural skin oils.

SYMPTOMS

Symptoms of dry skin include itching, flakiness, redness, and cracking.

REMEDIES

- Moisturize your skin with a lotion or cream, especially after bathing. Moisturizers keep water and oils in and dryness out. Use a lip balm to prevent or treat chapping of the lips.
- When showering or bathing, use cool water. Hot water coaxes oil from the pores. When bathing, put

EARS AND ALTITUDE

Do your ears begin popping as the plane takes off? The sudden change in altitude causes this sensation, which is an imbalance in air pressure in the middle ear. To reduce the discomfort:

- During takeoff, use a nasal decongestant. When nasal membranes swell, they interfere with the body's ability to adjust to changes in air pressure.
- Try chewing gum and swallowing a lot during the plane's takeoff and descent. If that doesn't work, try swallowing with your mouth closed and your nose pinched. This action will help draw pressure away from the middle ear.

The "popping" sensation can be a frightening and painful one for young children. Chewing gum or sucking on a lollipop may help relieve the pressure.

bath oil in the water. However, before adding the oil, immerse yourself in the water, advises James Shaw, M.D., chief of the division of dermatology at Good Samaritan Hospital in Portland, Oregon. After the water penetrates your skin, the oil you add will help seal it in. (If you add the oil first, it will adhere to your skin before the water has a chance to penetrate.)

- Use mild soaps containing oil, cream, or lanolin. Harsh soaps can contain lye, which removes oil and moisture along with the dirt.
- To counteract the drying effects of furnaces, fireplaces, stoves, and air conditioners, humidify your home and your work environment.
- Wear protective clothing when you're in the sun. Use a sunscreen with a sun protection factor (SPF) of 15 or more on exposed skin areas.
- Wear vinyl or latex gloves when handling kerosene or other chemicals or when washing dishes with harsh detergents.

Call your physician if dryness persists despite remedies or cracking skin becomes infected.

EAR INFECTIONS

Some old germs never die. They don't even fade away. Instead, they move from one site in the body to another, starting a new infection upon their arrival.

Such is the case with many ear infections. This is what happens: Suppose your child has an upper-respiratory infection—a cold, for example. After the illness has run its course, she is once again in high spirits and ready for a new adventure. Unfortunately, opportunistic germs in her throat feel the same way. Traveling through the Eustachian tube, like nomads, they migrate upward to the middle ear.

The symptoms of middle-ear infection, which doctors call *otitis media,* include earache, vomiting, diarrhea, and high fever. According to the National Center for Health Statistics, *otitis media* is the most common diagnosis in children under age 15. (Children under age 2 are at very high risk of developing *otitis media,* so parents should watch for symptoms. In particular, suspect an ear infection if an infant repeatedly touches or tugs at an ear.)

A middle-ear infection can lead to permanent hearing problems and, in rare cases, to meningitis (inflammation of brain tissue) and mastoiditis (inflammation of the bone behind the ear). If you suspect an ear infection, call a physician immediately. If a bacterial infection is present, your doctor can prescribe antibiotics and drain the ear if necessary. The duration of middle-ear infections varies. However, with prompt treatment, an infection will usually begin clearing up in just a few days.

Be aware that although middle-ear infections usually occur in children, they can sometimes afflict adults.

Therefore, if you have the symptoms of *otitis media,* you, too, should seek a physician's treatment.

CAUSES

Recent respiratory infections such as colds and flu, enlarged adenoids, diseased tonsils, allergies, and mumps and measles can all lead to ear infections.

SYMPTOMS

Symptoms of an ear infection include fluid buildup, earache, hearing impairment, leaking pus, vomiting, diarrhea, irritability, pulling at the ear (small children), and fever that can rise to as high as 105° F. Ear infections often awaken young children at night, causing them to cry out in pain. Sometimes fluid buildup occurs without other signs of infection, a condition known as noninfected middle-ear effusion.

REMEDIES

- Prop up the head with an extra pillow to help drain the eustachian tube.
- Avoid smoking. The smoke can cause congestion in the Eustachian tube.
- Use an over-the-counter drug, such as acetaminophen, to help relieve ear pain. Children and teenagers should not be given aspirin for an ear infection because of the risk of Reye syndrome, a rare but serious illness reported to be associated with taking aspirin.

- Ask your physician to recommend a nasal spray that will help relieve ear pressure and open the eustachian tube.
- Carefully follow your physician's instructions on the use of prescribed medications.

Note: Another, less serious, ear infection can also occur in children and adults. Often called "swimmer's ear," it develops in the outer ear—the canal that leads to the outside from the eardrum—and causes pain, slight fever, itching, hearing impairment, or discharges of pus. Swimming in polluted or chlorinated water is a common cause of this condition. Other causes include poor hygiene, irritation of the ear with swabs or ear plugs, and excessive moisture. This condition also requires the attention of a physician.

Call your physician if you or your child develop an ear infection; the fever exceeds 102°F despite remedies; severe headache, dizziness, or swelling around the ear develops; or the earache lasts longer than two days.

FLU

Influenza germs are smart. In order to infiltrate our bodies from year to year, they continually redesign themselves so that no single vaccine can remain effective against them. One year we have the Hong Kong flu. The next year, it's the Leningrad or Taiwan flu. The following year, it's an entirely different strain. Like a cold, influenza is a contagious upper-respiratory infection, but its symptoms—such as fever and cough—are more distressing. Usually it takes one to two weeks for the illness to run its course and for you to start feeling like yourself again.

CAUSES

The flu is caused by a viral infection. Your risk of getting the flu increases if you suffer from stress or fatigue, if your diet is poor, or if another illness has weakened your immune system.

SYMPTOMS

Symptoms include chills, fever, headache, runny nose, muscle aches, hoarseness, sore throat, and dry cough.

REMEDIES

- Get plenty of bed rest.
  - Drink plenty of liquids and eat chicken soup to help thin lung secretions and prevent dehydration.
    - Avoid milk. It can thicken lung secretions in some people, worsening lung congestion.
    - Use a vaporizer to ease congestion.
    - Take a pain reliever to help alleviate headache and muscle

Is it Really the Flu?

Did you know that the last time you had the stomach flu, it actually may have been a case of food poisoning? Sometimes bacteria present in food can produce toxins in your body. These toxins can cause acute inflammation of the intestines, which can trigger diarrhea, abdominal pain, and vomiting. The symptoms of food poisoning may not appear for hours or several days.

Most cases are mild, and symptoms last only a day or two. Notify your physician if your symptoms are severe or last longer than two days. The continued loss of fluids caused by vomiting and diarrhea could lead to serious dehydration. Your doctor may need to prescribe antibiotics—even hospitalization—to help cure your condition. The best means of avoiding food poisoning is proper hygiene and thorough cooking of foods.

aches and pains. Children and teenagers should not be given aspirin for a viral infection because of the risk of Reye syndrome, a rare but serious illness reported to be associated with aspirin.

- Gargle with salt water (1 teaspoon salt to a pint of water) to soothe a sore throat. Gargling with strong tea may also help.
- Use over-the-counter cough syrups, decongestants, and nasal sprays. Be aware that such medications can mask symptoms, however, so don't overexert yourself before you've really recovered.
- Don't smoke. Smoking will only worsen coughing.

Call your physician if your fever or cough worsens, you cough up blood or greenish or yellowish sputum, you are short of breath or have chest pain, or you have other unusual or worrisome symptoms.

HEADACHES

Headache pain may occur in one part of the head or all over the head. One of the most common causes of headaches is tightening of the muscles of the scalp, neck, face, and jaw. Stress and anxiety can trigger this response.

Serious underlying problems, such as a brain tumor or chronic high blood pressure, can also cause headaches. You should see a physician if you suffer from migraines or frequent or unexplained headaches.

CAUSES

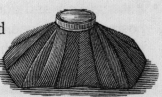

Headache pain can be caused by stress, anxiety, smoking, excess alcohol or caffeine consumption, caffeine withdrawal, adverse reactions to medications, fever, irregular eating patterns, sleeping problems, fatigue, eyestrain, sitting or lying in awkward positions that strain neck muscles, sinus infection, ear infection, toothache, eating meats containing sodium nitrites, hormonal changes, and a rapid rise in blood pressure as a result of anger, sexual excitement, or vigorous activity.

SYMPTOMS

Symptoms of a headache include pain in the front or back of the head, across the scalp, over the temples, or all over the head. The pain sometimes involves the neck and shoulders as well.

REMEDIES

- Take aspirin or acetaminophen to relieve the pain.
- Apply cold or warm compresses to the affected area.
- Massage shoulder and neck muscles.
- Don't smoke.
- Don't drink alcohol.
- Don't chew gum. Gum-chewing tenses muscles; tense muscles, in turn, can cause a headache.
- Stop sitting or lying in positions that may strain neck muscles.

- Eat regularly and don't skip meals. If you miss or postpone meals, your blood sugar could fall, causing blood vessels in the head to tighten. This condition can lead to a headache.
- Monitor caffeine consumption. If you drink three or four cups of caffeinated coffee each weekday and then don't drink coffee at all on the weekend, you could suffer a caffeine-withdrawal headache. Headaches may also result from drinking too much caffeine.
- Don't strain your eyes. If you wear eyeglasses, see that you have the correct prescription.
- If you suspect a prescription or nonprescription medication is causing your head pain, talk with your physician about taking an alternative medication.

Call your physician if your pain is noticeable only when you bend your neck or move around, your pain resulted from a head injury, your pain has no apparent cause, your headaches are becoming frequent, or your headache is accompanied by blurred vision or dizziness.

HEARTBURN

Heartburn is a burning sensation beneath the breastbone that often radiates to the neck and shoulders. The condition is sometimes accompanied by the regurgitation of a sour, bitter material into your throat or mouth. Heartburn is caused by acid reflux, which is the reverse flow of acid from the stomach to the esophagus, or food pipe.

High-fat foods and caffeinated beverages are common causes of heartburn because they relax the ring of muscle at the top of the stomach, called the lower esophageal sphincter. When the sphincter muscle becomes lazy, it allows acidic stomach contents to move back up the esophagus, causing heartburn.

CAUSES

Causes of heartburn include foods with a high fat or high acid content, effervescent drinks, aspirin and other drugs, hiatal hernia, and ulceration of the esophagus. Your risk of developing heartburn increases if you smoke, drink to excess, are overweight, are pregnant, or suffer from stress.

SYMPTOMS

Symptoms of heartburn include a burning sensation in the chest or abdomen, belching, bloating, regurgitation of stomach matter into your throat or mouth, and chest pain.

REMEDIES

- Using wood blocks, elevate the head of your bed at least 6 inches. The elevation assists gravity in keeping your stomach acids where they belong.
- Don't overeat.
- Don't lie down after large meals.

- Don't eat anything two to three hours before going to bed.
- Don't smoke. Cigarettes relax the lower esophageal sphincter and predispose you to heartburn.
- Decrease the amount of alcohol, chocolate, fats, and peppermints you consume. These substances may relax the lower esophageal sphincter.
- If you are overweight, shed the extra pounds. A leaner abdomen decreases the pressure on your stomach, which in turn may lessen reflux.
- Take an over-the-counter antacid to relieve occasional heartburn. Also, ask your pharmacist about a new therapy that combines antacids with an over-the-counter anti-ulcer medication to produce long-lasting relief.
- Chew gum. Gum-chewing increases saliva production. Saliva, in turn, neutralizes regurgitated acids.

Call your physician if you develop heartburn three or four times a week, you experience dizziness or shortness of breath, you experience nausea, you vomit blood, or you have difficulty swallowing.

HEMORRHOIDS

Hemorrhoids are clusters of veins located just under the membrane that lines the lowest part of the rectum and anus. There are four kinds of hemorrhoids: first-degree hemorrhoids, which remain inside the rectum at all times; second-degree hemorrhoids, which protrude out of the anal opening during bowel movements but return afterward; third-degree hemorrhoids, which protrude during bowel movements and remain there until pushed back; and fourth-degree hemorrhoids, which remain outside the anal opening.

According to the National Digestive Diseases Information Clearinghouse (NDDIC), one of every two Americans develops hemorrhoids by the age of 50. Hemorrhoids are especially common in pregnant women.

CAUSES

Stress, straining during bowel movements, heavy lifting, obesity, pregnancy, and prolonged sitting and standing can all cause hemorrhoids. Diet plays a major role in the development of hemorrhoids as well. A diet containing a high proportion of refined foods (rather than foods with natural roughage) increases the likelihood of constipation and, therefore, increases the likelihood of hemorrhoids.

SYMPTOMS

Symptoms of hemorrhoids include pain, itching, and a noticeable lump in the rectal or anal area that may bleed. Blood from hemorrhoids tends to be bright-red. (If you notice dark blood mixed with stools, see your physician. This may be symptom of a more serious condition.)

REMEDIES

- Eat at least 30 grams of fiber a day. Fiber promotes regular bowel movements and reduces straining. Among foods rich in fiber are fruits such as apples and prunes, vegetables such as broccoli and cauliflower, grains such as brown rice, and legumes such as beans and sweet peas. Bran cereals and whole-wheat bread are also good sources of fiber.
- Use relaxation techniques if you are suffering from stress (see page 39).
- If you are overweight, shed the extra pounds.
- After bowel movements, clean the anal area with soft, moistened, non-colored, and non-perfumed toilet paper.
- Avoid scratching hemorrhoids. Doing so can cause further damage. Over-the-counter preparations cannot cure hemorrhoids, but they can help relieve itching and swelling.
- To relieve discomfort, sit in a warm bath.

Call your physician if your hemorrhoids cause you severe pain, bleeding is excessive or blood is dark, or you develop a fourth-degree hemorrhoid.

INSOMNIA

Most folks regard interruptions of sleep as a source of frustration, especially when sleeplessness extends from late-night television to the rooster's early crow.

Insomnia can result from a long list of causes—the most common of which often stem from stress and anxiety. For many people, insomnia lasts only a day or two. For others, insomnia may seem to last indefinitely.

CAUSES

Causes of insomnia include stress, anxiety, depression, painful illness, shortness of breath, hot weather, noise, irregular work hours, jet lag, smoking, drinking alcoholic or caffeinated beverages, frequent urination, drug reactions, lack of exercise, and an uncomfortable sleeping environment.

SYMPTOMS

Symptoms of insomnia include irritability, fatigue, and the inability to fall sleep—or stay asleep—at night.

REMEDIES

- Keep regular sleep hours. If a can't-be-missed television movie starts at midnight, program the VCR to record it, and tune into your dreams instead.
- Arise at the same time each morning, even after nights of little sleep. Regular sleeping habits help build successful sleeping patterns in the long run.
- Use relaxation techniques to alleviate stress or anxiety (see page 39).
- Make your sleeping environment as comfortable as possible. Plump pillows, a supportive mattress, and cozy sheets and blankets can work wonders.

- Don't smoke. Cravings for nicotine can awaken you several times during the night.
- Don't drink large amounts of any beverage. If you do, it's guaranteed you'll be walking back and forth to the bathroom all night long.
- Limit your alcohol intake or, better yet, avoid alcohol altogether. After its initial calming effect wears off, an alcoholic beverage tends to awaken you.
- Avoid eating a big meal right before going to bed. Your whole body needs to go to sleep, including your stomach.
- Get plenty of exercise during the day or early evening. When bedtime arrives, your body will be ready for sleep.
- Read a book or listen to relaxing music just before going to bed. Reading can make your eyelids heavy; music can calm your spirit.
- If you are tossing and turning, do not try to force sleep. While you're awake, relax: Read a book or write a letter. When you're too tired to stay awake, go back to bed and try to sleep again.

Call your physician if your insomnia may be due to depression, stress, or anxiety; you suspect your insomnia is a reaction to a medication you're taking; or your insomnia becomes chronic.

LARYNGITIS

Imagine this: You're the odds-on favorite to win the hog-calling contest at the county fair. But when the big day arrives and you're finally on the stage of the bandshell waving to your fans, you open your mouth and nothing comes out.

The word laryngitis can strike fear into the hearts of those who depend on their voices for a living. Laryngitis is an inflammation of the mucous membrane lining the voice box, or larynx, which is located in the upper part of the respiratory tract. Laryngitis can cause hoarseness and temporary loss of speech.

CAUSES

Laryngitis may result from a bacterial or viral infection, such as a cold or the flu; from an irritation of the mucous membrane of the larynx, such as that caused by smoking; or from overuse of the voice. It may also stem from tonsillitis, tuberculosis, the early stages of some forms of cancer, or paralysis of the vocal cords. Chronic or persistent laryngitis is most often caused by smoking, air pollution, or dust.

SYMPTOMS

Sore throat, inflammation in the throat, temporary loss of speech, hoarseness, slight fever, dryness, scratchiness, and a feeling that you have a lump in your throat are all symptoms of laryngitis. In rare instances, difficulty with swallowing can occur.

REMEDIES

- Quit smoking and don't drink alcoholic beverages.
- Rest the voice until the laryngitis subsides. Don't even whisper. Communicate with notes or sign language instead.
- Avoid coughing, which can prolong hoarseness. If necessary, use an over-the-counter medication to suppress coughing.
- Use a cool-mist humidifier; it will moisten the vocal cords and reduce irritation of the mucous membranes. You can also breathe in steam to achieve the same effect.
- Take an over-the-counter pain reliever, if desired, to alleviate throat soreness.
- Check your air conditioner. The filter could be a source of molds and pollutants that can irritate your larynx.

Call your physician if your laryngitis persists more than one week without improvement, you cough up blood, you have difficulty swallowing or breathing, or you have a high fever.

MIGRAINE

Dictionaries list "misery," "torment," and "torture" as synonyms for "agony." To sufferers of migraine, you'd need all of those words, and perhaps a few more, to describe the pain.

One theory about migraines is that they occur when the blood vessels in the head expand and press on nerve fibers, causing pain. Another theory is that migraines result from the blood vessels constricting and thus blocking blood flow to parts of the brain; this may cause the visual impairment and numbness that often accompany or precede a migraine headache. The blood vessels then become full of blood and press on surrounding nerves, causing pain.

Migraine headaches may occur as many as several times in one week or as few as one or two times every two or three years, according to the National Institute of Neurological Disorders and Stroke. The duration of migraines varies from a few minutes to several days. A classic migraine headache generally lasts one or two days. Migraine headaches occur more commonly in women than in men.

CAUSES

Causes of migraine may include stress, anxiety, fatigue, menstruation, adverse reactions to drugs, alcohol, bright lights, weather changes, altitude, and certain foods, including the following: red wine, champagne, cheese, hot dogs, salami, bacon, ham, pickled herring, chicken livers, chocolate, cocoa, homemade yeast bread, yogurt, buttermilk, sour cream, ice cream, mincemeat, apples, lentils, peas, beans, apricots, cherries, figs, peaches, pears, raisins, soy sauce, overripe bananas, meat tenderizer, and canned soup.

SYMPTOMS

A warning sensation, or aura, may indicate an approaching migraine. Individuals may experience blurred vision; smell unusual odors; or see flashing lights, zig-zag patterns, or wavy lines.

Symptoms of migraine include incapacitating pain on one or both sides of the head. Nausea, vomiting, diarrhea, tingling, numbness, weakness, dizziness, pain around one eye, droopy eyelids, and coordination problems may accompany the pain. Migraine sufferers may also become irritable and depressed.

Cluster headaches, a form of migraine most commonly experienced by men, occur in groups of up to six a day; episodes can last for weeks or months. Their chief symptom is intense pain on one side of the head, accompanied by tearing of the eye and a runny nose on the same side. Drinking and smoking may aggravate these headaches.

REMEDIES

- At the first sign of impending migraine, take an over-the-counter medication, such as aspirin or acetaminophen.
- If you suffer frequent migraines, try an herb called feverfew. The herb may take up to six weeks to achieve its full effect, but if taken daily it relieves pain in most cases. Available in tablet form, feverfew has no known serious side effects (see Feverfew, page 134).

- Apply a soft ice pack to the head. Use a towel to contain the ice.
- Rest in a quiet, dark room.
- Use relaxation techniques to reduce stress (see page 39).
- Don't smoke. The carbon monoxide in cigarettes can affect the flow of blood to the brain.
- Shield your eyes against bright lights or sunlight.
- Treatment and prevention of migraine sometimes consists of a drug-therapy program. Carefully follow your physician's instructions if he or she prescribes medication.
- Ask your physician about receiving drug injections if your migraines do not respond to oral medications.
- To prevent future migraines, avoid foods and beverages that seem to trigger your migraines. To identify the offending foods, keep a food diary.

Call your physician if your migraine causes extreme pain, the migraine pain persists for several days, or your migraines become more frequent.

NOSEBLEEDS

Let's face it, some things in life are unpredictable, and a nosebleed is one of them. Why does the nose suddenly decide to bleed? Is a nosebleed a sign of a serious problem? What's the best way to stop a nosebleed and prevent it from recurring?

Most of the time, a nosebleed is nothing to worry about. Did you know that something as simple as a sneeze can cause one? So can low humidity. Without adequate moisture, sensitive nose membranes may become dry and crack, opening tiny fissures. In addition, aging can thin nose membranes, making them vulnerable to rupture and bleeding. In some instances, however, a nosebleed can be a symptom of an underlying condition, such as high blood pressure, leukemia, liver disease, or a tumor. If you suffer from frequent nosebleeds, see your doctor.

CAUSES

Causes of nosebleed include dry air, blowing the nose too hard, sinus infection, nasal infection, injury, a change in atmospheric pressure, an underlying condition (including high blood pressure, leukemia, liver disease, typhoid fever, malaria, hardening of the arteries, hemophilia, or a tumor), and the use of certain drugs (including aspirin, oral contraceptives, and anticlotting medications).

SYMPTOMS

Symptoms of nosebleed include bright red blood if the bleeding occurs in the front of the nose, dark or bright red blood if the bleeding occurs in the back, lightheadedness if there is a significant loss of blood, and shortness of breath or rapid heartbeat if there is a major loss of blood.

REMEDIES

- Sit down and tilt your head forward to prevent blood backup from gagging you.
- Pinch your nose for five minutes or more to dam and stop the bleeding.
- When the bleeding stops, do not blow your nose for at least 24 hours. You've got to allow time for a solid clot to form.
- If the bleeding doesn't stop quickly, pinch the fleshy part of the nose for ten minutes more and apply an ice pack to the bridge of the nose.
- If the bleeding was caused by an injury, be gentle when you pinch the nose and be sure to apply ice.
- If the nosebleed continues after 30 minutes, or if you are bleeding heavily, seek medical treatment.
- To prevent nosebleeds, don't blow your nose like a trumpet. If you think a drug might be causing nosebleeds, ask your physician whether you can stop taking the drug or whether you can substitute another one.

Call your physician if your nosebleeds are frequent, your nosebleeds are very heavy or difficult to control, or you suspect a medication you are taking or an underlying illness such as high blood pressure could be responsible for your nosebleeds.

NAUSEA AND VOMITING

Nausea is that queasy feeling you get in your stomach when something isn't quite right down there. Sometimes vomiting is your body's way of remedying the problem, occurring when contracting stomach muscles force the stomach contents upward and out.

Nausea and vomiting are symptoms of a wide variety of illnesses, conditions, and reactions to physical or mental irritants. Provided your symptoms are not the result of serious illness, they should disappear in a day or two.

CAUSES

Nausea and vomiting can be induced by stomach infections, food poisoning, overeating, alcohol abuse, smoking, stress, anxiety, morning sickness in pregnancy, motion sickness, foul odors, and certain medications.

SYMPTOMS

Upset stomach, chills, sweating, headache, rapid heartbeat, and fever are all symptoms of nausea.

REMEDIES

- If your symptoms are due to stomach irritants—for example, a virus, spoiled food, or alcohol—let vomiting run its course. The sooner you get the offending substance out of your body, the sooner you will start to feel better.

- Don't drink alcoholic beverages or smoke if you feel nauseous. Both can irritate the stomach further.
- After vomiting stops, drink clear fluids such as water, tea, and bouillon to prevent dehydration, advises Cornelius P. Dooley, M.D., a gastroenterologist in Santa Fe, New Mexico.
- Avoid eating until you think your stomach can handle it.
- When you're ready to eat, choose easy-to-digest low-fat foods such as crackers, toast (unbuttered), gelatin, bananas, and applesauce. If your stomach is accepting, you may graduate to such foods as broiled fish, lean beef, and cottage cheese.
- If your nausea is due to motion sickness, take an over-the-counter product, such as Dramamine, to relieve it. If you're aboard a ship, you can obtain the medication at the ship's pharmacy or from the ship's doctor.

Call your physician if your symptoms persist for more than two days, you have severe abdominal pain, or you have a high fever or notice blood in your vomit.

RASH

Common rashes include those caused by dermatitis, eczema, hives, and heat. Dermatitis causes itching, redness, and swelling as a result of exposure to an irritant. For example, in contact dermatitis—one of several kinds of dermatitis—the skin breaks out after coming into contact with such irritants as poison ivy, detergents, cleansers, solvents, and insecticides. Sunburn and repeated exposure to hot water can increase your risk of developing contact dermatitis. Symptoms include itching, redness, and cracking of the skin.

Eczema causes itching, blistering, and thickening of the skin due to an allergic reaction to foods such as eggs or milk, to materials such as wool, or to lotions and creams. Stress and sweating can also increase your vulnerability to eczema.

Hives are itching welts that can be caused by an allergic reaction to food, drugs, and insect bites as well as emotional stress, sunlight, and heat and cold. Most of the time, hives are no cause for concern. However, in some people, the hives may be part of anaphylaxis, a severe allergic reaction that may hamper breathing and threaten the life of the victim. In rare instances, hives may also be associated with a serious underlying illness, such as hepatitis or cancer.

Heat rash causes tiny blisters and pimples that itch and burn. The rash develops when high temperatures, humidity, sunburn, fever, or tight clothing hamper the evaporation of sweat from the skin.

How long does a rash last? That depends on its cause and your treatment. Rashes caused by poison ivy, poison oak, or poison sumac usually disappear within two weeks. Eczema rashes usually disappear after their cause is eliminated. Hives may disappear within hours or stick around for days; eliminating or avoiding the cause reduces the risk of another outbreak, however. Heat rash will disappear after you learn to keep your cool.

Be aware that rashes can occur as part of chicken pox, measles, and many other viral or bacterial infections in which fever is usually a symptom. Contact your physician if you or a family member develops such an infection.

CAUSES

Rashes are caused by exposure to irritants such as poison ivy, poison oak, and poison sumac; various chemicals; various metals in wristwatches, earrings, and necklaces; allergic reactions to foods; certain medications; certain fabrics; insect stings and bites; stress and anxiety; and hot, humid weather.

SYMPTOMS

Redness, itching, burning, swelling, and cracking of the skin are all symptoms of a rash.

REMEDIES

- Apply cool, wet compresses to skin to relieve itching.
- To gain further relief, use an over-the-counter medication designed specifically for your condition.

- Don't scratch. You could further irritate your skin or cause an infection.
- To avoid irritating the skin and prevent further outbreaks of heat rash, eczema, or hives, wear soft, loose-fitting clothing.
- If you have eczema, avoid wearing clothing made of wool or polyester.
- When bathing, use lukewarm water and non-soap cleansers.
- If you don't know which allergen is provoking your skin rash, keep a diary. In it, note the foods you eat or the objects with which you come in contact daily. When you develop a rash, refer to your diary and try to pinpoint the cause.

Note: Get emergency treatment if you have hives and any of the following symptoms:
- Shortness of breath
- Swollen lips
- Tightness in the throat

Call your physician if you develop a rash of unknown origin, the skin becomes infected, or you develop a fever or other symptoms of viral or bacterial infection.

SPRAINS AND STRAINS

It's the farm bowl, and it's your moment of glory. As you race through the potato field, the football tucked between chest and forearm, you elude tacklers with the grace of a gazelle. The result? A touchdown—and a pulled muscle.

Most of us have pulled up lame on occasion because of a strain or sprain suffered during a softball game, a tennis match, or even a romp in the yard with children.

A strain, or pulled muscle, occurs when a muscle stretches beyond its limits. In some cases, the muscle may tear or even rupture. If the strain results from sudden movement—a twist or a turn—you will experience severe pain at first, then tenderness and swelling. Bruises may appear after several days. If the strain results from overuse over a long period of time—that is, if it is chronic—you will experience soreness and tenderness several hours after the activity.

A sprain occurs when a ligament connecting a muscle to a bone tears. A tear may be mild or moderate, or it may be severe, causing a complete rupture. Sprains produce tenderness at first. Within hours, swelling, severe pain, black and blue discoloration, and limited mobility or disability occur.

Sprains and strains usually heal in two to four weeks. If the injury does not involve loss of mobility, it may not require a physician's treatment. Those sprains involving a rupture may require surgical treatment, however. When in doubt about the severity of an injury, call your physician.

CAUSES

Causes of strains and sprains include sudden twists and turns, overstretching, lifting, and bending.

SYMPTOMS

Pain, tenderness, swelling, stiffness, skin discoloration, and loss of mobility are all symptoms of sprains and strains.

REMEDIES

- If you have a severely injured ankle, don't walk on it. Have someone help you from the scene. If you have a severe wrist or shoulder injury, have someone place your arm in a sling.
- Use the RICE treatment. RICE is an acronym for Rest, Ice, Compression, and Elevation. Here's what to do:
  1. Rest the injured part of the body.
  2. Ice should be applied to the affected area.
  3. Compress the injury with an elastic bandage or a cloth.
  4. Elevate the injured part above the heart.

Continue applying ice to the injured area for 20 minutes every two hours to ease pain and reduce swelling. After 48 hours, you may substitute heat treatments. To apply heat, soak the injured area in hot water or apply hot compresses. Keep the injured part elevated to allow fluid to drain, thereby reducing swelling. Use aspirin or ibuprofen to relieve pain.

Call your physician if your injury or your pain is severe or if swelling and discoloration of the affected area continue to worsen even after you follow these treatment guidelines.

SORE THROAT

If your physician has diagnosed you with pharyngitis, don't worry. You needn't make out a will just yet. Pharyngitis simply means sore throat. If your sore throat is the result of postnasal drip or if it accompanies symptoms of the flu or a cold, then you can probably treat it yourself. Most sore throats clear up in two to six days.

CAUSES

Causes of sore throat include bacterial, viral, and fungal infections; fatigue; smoking; postnasal drip; breathing through the mouth; dry air; air pollution; excessive coughing; and tooth and gum infections.

SYMPTOMS

Symptoms of sore throat include throat pain, difficulty swallowing, fever, swollen glands, appetite loss, headache, and red, swollen throat tissue.

REMEDIES

- Gargle with salt water (1 teaspoon salt to a pint of water) or strong tea. Suck on lozenges or hard candy to keep the throat moist.
- Drink plenty of fluids to lubricate the throat and prevent further irritation.
- Try eating raw garlic. Some studies indicate that garlic can help fight infection.
- Use a cool-mist humidifier to further relieve dryness of the throat.

Call your physician if your sore throat is accompanied by a high fever, swollen glands, chills, fatigue, or pain that intensifies when you swallow.

SUNBURN

While down at the river, you're having so much fun splashing in the inner tube that you lose track of the time. Later, as you towel off and get ready for the trip home, you notice the burning pain all over.

"You look like a lobster," someone comments.

And you feel like a fool. After all, a sunburn, you're well aware, can put you at higher risk of developing skin cancer. You should have used a sunscreen. You should have worn a hat. You should have limited your time in the sun.

But you didn't, and now your skin is red and swollen, and you're in pain. If the burn is severe enough to cause blistering, nausea, and vomiting, you should see a physician.

Next time, when outside in the sun, cover your skin with loose-fitting, light-colored clothes made of loose-weave fabrics, and wear a hat. And don't forget sunscreen, available in oil, cream, paste, or liquid. It's probably best to use a sunscreen with a sun protection factor (SPF) of at least 15. Reapply your sunscreen frequently when out-of-doors.

Individuals who should be especially wary of the sun include those with a family history of skin cancer; those who burn easily; outdoor workers; pregnant women; and persons taking tranquilizers, diuretics, antihistamines, and antibiotics, all of which increase the skin's sensitivity to the sun.

CAUSES

Sunburn is caused by overexposure to the ultraviolet rays of the sun, which are strongest between 10 A.M. and 3 P.M. Sunlamps can also cause severe damage to the skin.

SYMPTOMS

Symptoms of sunburn may sometimes include pain, redness, swelling, soreness, and blistering of the skin; nausea and vomiting; diarrhea; fever; and chills.

REMEDIES

- Apply cool compresses to the affected area. When the compresses become warm, wet them again and reapply. Continue the application for approximately 15 minutes. Repeat the procedure several times throughout the day.
- Take cool baths and drink plenty of water to restore fluids.
- If a blister is causing extreme pressure and discomfort, puncture it with a sterilized needle. But don't peel away the skin. Leave it in place; it protects the underlying skin against infection. Apply a skin cream containing aloe vera to reddened skin around the blister.

Call your physician if your sunburn causes severe blistering; if, in addition to sunburn, you experience nausea, vomiting, or diarrhea; if your body temperature reaches 101°F or more; or if pain and fever from sunburn continue for more than two days.

TOOTHACHE

On the second day of your family camping trip at Lake Cheerful, you awaken to a wonderful morning. The sun is out, the birds are chirping, and the smell of frying bacon—compliments of your early-rising spouse—fills the air. As you breathe in the aromas of bacon and fresh country air, you notice the ache in your mouth.

DENTAL EMERGENCIES

A fall or direct blow to the mouth can cause serious injury to the teeth and nearby tissues. Knowing the right way to handle a dental emergency can mean the difference between saving or losing a tooth.

The American Dental Association recommends the following tips on what to do in case of a knocked-out tooth:

- If the tooth is dirty, rinse it gently in running water.
- Do not scrub it or remove any attached tissue fragments.
- Gently insert and hold the tooth in its socket. If this is not possible, place the tooth in a cup of cool water.
- This is a dental emergency. Go to your dentist immediately (within 30 minutes if possible).

Could it be the beginning of a toothache? Naw. That's impossible.

At breakfast, you toast everyone with a glass of cold orange juice as you look forward to the day's events: a hike, a canoe trip, and a marshmallow roast. And then you drink.

The pain is excruciating. Was it the coldness of the orange juice or the sweetness? Who knows. What matters is that you're in agony, and you're 100 miles from civilization and the nearest dentist.

Toothaches always seem to occur at the worst times—on weekends, in the middle of the night, or when you're camping at Lake Cheerful. The symptoms—including throbbing pain and inflammation of gums—are commonly the result of tooth decay.

But if your dentist recommends pulling your tooth, don't be too quick to agree. According to Walter J. Loesche, D.M.D, Ph.D., professor of dentistry and microbiology at the University of Michigan School of Dentistry, seven out of ten teeth classified as "hopeless" can actually be saved by cleaning out the infection and applying antimicrobial medication. If you think you need a second opinion, your dentist can probably give you pain medication to tide you over while you seek out another's advice.

CAUSES

Decay is a common cause of toothache. But toothaches can also develop as a result of sinus problems, ear infections, tooth injury (such as chipping), and, in rare instances, chest pain related to heart problems.

SYMPTOMS

Symptoms of toothache include pain, aching, sensitivity to sugar, sensitivity to heat and cold, and inflammation and swelling of the gums.

REMEDIES

- Rinse the mouth with lukewarm water to remove trapped food particles that could be causing the pain.
- Use oil of cloves—available at any pharmacy—to provide temporary relief. This is an old remedy, but it works. Using a wad of cotton saturated with the diluted oil, apply the remedy to the tooth (see Oil of Cloves, page 143), being careful to avoid the gums.
- Take aspirin or acetaminophen. (Do not apply the aspirin directly to the affected area, however; it could burn the gums.)
- If you have swelling, place a cold compress against the cheek over the affected tooth for 10 or 15 minutes. Repeat throughout the day.
- Avoid using the affected tooth when chewing.
- Avoid sugary foods and drinks.
- Make a dental appointment as soon as possible.

Call your physician if your toothache is accompanied by chest pain, your tooth pain could be caused by an ear or sinus infection, or you have unusual symptoms.

URINARY TRACT INFECTIONS

Painful, annoying urinary tract infections are caused by bacteria in any part of your urinary tract, including your kidneys, ureters (the tubes that carry urine to the bladder from the kidneys), urethra (the tube that empties the bladder when you urinate), or bladder (the sac that holds the urine before it is released through the urethra).

Although men also can suffer from urinary tract infections, women are much more likely to get them. Because a woman's urethra is shorter than a man's, bacteria can more easily reach the bladder. Also, because the urethra is closer to the rectum on a woman's body, bacteria from the rectum can more easily travel to the urinary tract.

With appropriate antibiotic treatment, symptoms of a urinary tract infection can disappear within days. However, patients need to continue taking medication for ten days or so to make certain all traces of bacteria have been eradicated.

CAUSES

Urinary tract infections are sometimes caused by bacteria migrating from the intestines to the urethra. Sometimes an enlarged prostate gland in men and pregnancy in women cause an infection by restricting the flow of urine from the bladder, allowing urine to collect and bacteria to multiply. Sexual intercourse and the use of a catheter (tube) to drain the bladder can also be sources of infection.

SYMPTOMS

Symptoms of urinary tract infection include pain, burning, frequent urination, an urge to urinate even when the bladder contains little urine, bloody or foul-smelling urine, cloudy urine, yellowish-green urine, abdominal or lower-back pain, and fever and chills.

REMEDIES

- Drink lots of water to flush out bacteria. This remedy not only helps treat urinary tract infections, but also helps prevent them in the first place.
- On occasion, substitute cranberry juice for water. Some evidence suggests that this juice inhibits bacterial growth.
- Always keep the anal and genital areas clean to prevent bacteria buildup and the risk of recurrent infection.
- When you have an urge to urinate, do so. Holding in urine risks a buildup of bacteria.
- Urinate after sexual intercourse to help wash away bacteria.
- After bowel movements, wipe from front to back to prevent bacteria from reaching the urethra.
- Don't use scented douches, washes, or hygiene sprays. They can irritate the urethra.

Call your physician if you have a urinary tract infection. You will need a prescription drug or another physician's remedy to cure the infection. You should also call your doctor if your temperature rises to 101°F or more after two days of treatment; you have blood in your urine; your condition does not improve within a week; you believe your symptoms may be caused by a condition other than a urinary tract infection, such as a sexually transmitted disease; or you believe the infection has spread to your kidneys. Shaking chills and aching in the lower back are symptoms of kidney infection, a serious condition called pyelonephritis.

VARICOSE VEINS

If you have varicose veins, you're not alone: Over 40 million other Americans also have them. Varicose veins are swollen, stretched veins in the legs, close to the surface of the skin, caused by increased pressure of the blood in the veins.

Because blood from the legs must return to the heart uphill, against the force of gravity, the veins in the legs have one-way valves to prevent blood from flowing back down toward the feet. But when the veins are stretched from pressure or when the valves are injured in some way, the valves cannot close properly, and some blood travels back down. When the blood accumulates in pools, the veins are stretched even more, and varicose veins are formed.

VEIN WATCH

Are varicose veins harmful to your health? Not usually. But here's what to do if complications do occur:

- Ulcers can develop if blood flow to the tissues of the leg is hampered. If a patch of brownish skin or a sore develops on or near a varicose vein, see your doctor.

- The swollen veins can bleed profusely if bumped or cut—a situation that requires immediate medical attention.

- Thrombophlebitis, or simple phlebitis, occurs when a clot forms in a vein, causing inflammation and swelling. If such a problem develops, your physician may prescribe anticlotting drugs and you may need to be hospitalized; you may even need surgery. Your doctor may suggest daily medication—usually aspirin—to prevent clots from forming.

CAUSES

Varicose veins are caused by a number of factors that put excess pressure on the veins in the legs: prolonged sitting, especially when the legs are crossed; prolonged standing; lack of exercise; confining clothes; obesity (which puts excess pressure on the legs); heredity (a tendency toward weak vein walls and valves); and height (tall people may be more susceptible to varicose veins because their blood needs to travel farther in its trip back up to the heart).

Women are more likely to have varicose veins than men, largely due to hormonal factors. Pregnancy accentuates this difference because special hormones released during this time tend to relax the walls of the veins. Also, varicose veins often appear during the last few months of pregnancy due to the increased strain on the woman's legs from the weight of the growing fetus. These veins may recede, however, after the birth of the baby.

SYMPTOMS

Varicose veins are very noticeable because they form close to the skin. They appear as bulging, bluish, cord-like lines running down the legs. Symptoms that accompany varicose veins are feelings of achiness, heaviness, and fatigue in the legs, especially at the end of the day. Itchy, scaly skin often covers the affected areas. In advanced cases, swollen ankles and leg cramps can occur.

REMEDIES

- Exercise to promote blood circulation and to keep leg muscles fit. You don't have to run marathons—walking, riding a bike, or using the gym's stair machine will do.
- Wear elastic stockings, available from medical-supply stores in waist-high, thigh-high, and knee-high sizes. The pressure they exert will help keep blood from pooling.
- If you are obese, lose weight. When you are over-weight, your vessels are under greater strain because they must carry more blood, says Luis Navarro, M.D., author of *No More Varicose Veins*.
- If you work standing up, spend your breaks sitting down with your legs elevated to promote blood flow.
- Avoid crossing your legs, which restricts blood flow.
- Avoid wearing tight-fitting clothing, such as panty hose with elastic tops.
- If you don't have breathing problems, elevate the foot of your bed a few inches to promote circulation overnight.
- Eat a well-balanced diet in order to keep your muscles and circulatory system operating at optimum levels.
- If you need to thin your blood to reduce the risk of clot formation, consider eating garlic and taking vitamin E. Both garlic and vitamin E are blood-thinners. (Check with your doctor first before trying this treatment.)

Call your physician if you have excessive pain, you cut a varicose vein and it bleeds profusely, or you want to remove or shrink your varicose veins. Physicians can inject agents that can collapse or shrivel enlarged veins. They can also perform surgery that strips them away or use a new pulse-light therapy that heats and destroys varicose veins.

WARTS

Witches aren't the only people who get warts. Ordinary folks get them too.

Actually, the right word is "catch," not "get," because warts are contagious, the spawn of a mischievous virus. Like colds and flu, they spread from person to person.

Warts are infectious growths in the outer layers of the skin. Most warts have a rough surface and may be flat or bumpy. Warts are caused by exposure to any of more than 30 viruses that can remain inactive for up to six months after contact. Warts can occur practically anywhere, sometimes in clusters—on the scalp, face, neck, back, hands, wrists, and knees; on the bottom of the feet; and in the genital areas (rectum, penis, and vaginal entrance).

Genital warts may grow in pink or red clusters resembling cauliflower, and they are more contagious than other warts. Usually, the warts spread by sexual contact.

Plantar warts grow on the soles of the feet. These warts cause considerable pain because the tissue swelling pushes inward with the pressure of each step; the discomfort from plantar warts feels like walking with a pebble in your shoe.

Warts can take several months to develop. And while some of them disappear in a month or two, others may remain for several years, resisting repeated efforts to eradicate them. Besides, elimination of warts is no guarantee that they won't return. You may use home remedies on warts that occur on most parts of your body, but only a physician should treat genital warts.

CAUSES

Warts are caused by any of 35 different viruses. Genital warts are usually spread via sexual contact.

SYMPTOMS

Warts may feel tender or itchy. Their size and shape vary depending on the location and severity of the viral infection.

REMEDIES

In the case of genital warts, see your doctor. Otherwise:

- Wait. Many warts are like spoiled children demanding attention: If you ignore them, they may go away.
- Apply an over-the-counter preparation containing salicylic acid and lactic acid. It can erode the wart, en-

abling you to peel it away. To avoid irritating the surrounding skin, make sure you follow the label instructions carefully.

- Apply castor oil twice a day. Its acid content may disintegrate the wart.
- Use brain power. There is evidence to suggest that warts will disappear if you believe they will. It's a matter of mind over warts. Try hypnosis or self-hypnosis. Martin Young, Ph.D., a psychologist at the University of Massachusetts Medical Center at Worcester, says hypnosis enables patients to lower their skin temperature. "If you create cold, you decrease the blood flow, potentially starving the virus that causes the wart." Patients can learn self-hypnosis techniques from licensed health professionals.
- If you have a plantar wart that really smarts, see your doctor. In the meanwhile, comfort it with soft pads and try an over-the-counter medication to relieve pain.
- To avoid spreading warts to other parts of your body, do not scratch them. Wash your hands after touching the warts.
- If home remedies fail, a physician can cut, burn, or freeze the warts away.

Call your physician if you can't identify the growth, the wart is causing you pain, the wart area becomes infected, or the wart is located in the genital area.

MEDICINE CHEST

Today we have vaccines to protect ourselves from measles, chicken pox, and whooping cough. But if you grew up in the first half of this century, you may recall that these vaccines were not available—there were no instant cures.

On the second or third day of your illness, the doctor would show up at your door with his black bag bulging with the essentials of the healing art: a stethoscope, a "Say ah" stick, and a tiny hammer with which to strike your kneecaps. And let's not forget the wide variety of medicines he brought that could be swallowed or rubbed on.

Many of the following remedies may bring back childhood memories. Others may be new to you. Just remember, these remedies aren't meant to replace a doctor's care. So if you have suspicious or worrisome symptoms, give your doctor a call.

ALOE VERA

Farmers, lumberjacks, anglers, and hunters—all of whom get roughed up by everything from thorns and splinters to barbed wire and fish hooks—are among those who ought to keep aloe vera close by.

Aloe vera is a plant of the lily family native to Africa. Its secret lies in two ingredients: salicylates—the same anti-inflammatory agents found in aspirin—and mag-

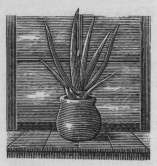

nesium lactate—an ingredient that inhibits skin reactions that cause itching. You can buy skin creams and gels containing aloe vera at your local pharmacy. But you might find that aloe vera taken directly from the plant itself works best for treating minor skin damage.

Treatment: Buy an aloe vera plant at your local plant nursery or garden shop. Slit one of its leaves lengthwise, squeeze out the gel, and apply the gel directly to the injury site. Apply the gel five or six times a day until the affected area heals.

Warning: Some people are allergic to aloe vera. If you develop a rash, stop using it. Do not ingest aloe vera; it should not be used to treat indigestion, constipation, or other internal conditions. Call your physician if you have a puncture wound or a serious burn.

CHAMOMILE

For centuries, people have used the aromatic perennial herb chamomile to treat a variety of conditions, including wounds, burns, colic, fever, and skin conditions. Dozens of studies have supported chamomile's traditional use as a digestive aid. (Several chemicals in chamomile appear to have a relaxing effect on the smooth muscle lining of the digestive tract.)

The plant has feathery green leaves and flowers with yellow centers and white petals. The herb grows in abundance in meadows and along roadsides in North America. Generally recognized as safe, chamomile is approved as an over-the-counter drug in Canada and is used in Europe in many over-the-counter preparations such as ointments, lotions, throat sprays, hair rinses, and inhalants.

In the U.S., commercial chamomile is available mostly in the form of tea that can be used to treat stomach pain and indigestion. You can buy chamomile tea in any supermarket. If you grow your own chamomile, you can make the tea yourself.

Treatment: To make chamomile tea, first dry the flower heads, then crush them. Next, place 2 teaspoons of the crushed flowers in a cup of boiling water. Steep for 10 minutes. Drink up to 3 cups a day.

Warning: In general, chamomile poses no health threat. If you have suffered previous anaphylactic shock reactions from ragweed, however, talk to your doctor about using the herb. If you are pregnant, do not use large amounts of this herb without first consulting your doctor. Excessive amounts of chamomile have been shown to cause nausea and vomiting in some people.

CHICKEN SOUP

Medical textbooks generally don't list chicken soup as a cold remedy. Nevertheless, it has been used for that purpose for many centuries—and to good effect.

The main benefit of chicken soup is that it helps clear congested nasal passages by promoting the flow of mucus. Chicken soup also replenishes lost body fluids and helps to relieve throat pain and swelling.

Treatment: Use a recipe of your choice to make your chicken-soup remedy. When making homemade soup, remove the chicken's skin before boiling to lower the fat and cholesterol content. (Always make sure the chicken is thoroughly cooked before serving. Under-cooked chicken may contain live salmonella bacteria, which can cause a serious infection of the digestive tract.) As the soup simmers, remember to keep the pot covered to prevent evaporation.

CRANBERRY JUICE

Cranberry juice not only prevents urinary tract infections, but it may cure them as well. How does it work? Some researchers believe cranberry juice creates an acid in the urine that kills the bacteria that cause bladder infections. Others believe that an ingredient in cranberry juice prevents germs from clinging to the bladder walls. Whether or not you believe in the cranberry cure, it may still be worth a try. At the very least, the juice will help you meet your daily requirement for vitamin C.

Treatment: Begin drinking cranberry juice at the first sign of a urinary tract infection. If you've developed urinary tract infections in the past, try drinking cranberry juice as a preventive measure. HINT: Because many cranberry juices available on store shelves contain high amounts of sugar, try taking cranberry juice in sugar-free tablet form.

Warning: If you have the symptoms of a urinary tract infection, see your doctor. Besides drinking cranberry juice to help fight and cure the infection, you may need to take antibiotics as well.

EPSOM SALTS

In the town of Epsom, England, in 1618, a substance called magnesium sulfate was found in abundance in spring water. Since that time, this substance—which we know today as Epsom salts—has been a favorite remedy for aching feet.

When added to water, Epsom salts help reduce foot swelling and soreness by drawing out sweat from the pores. Some doctors claim Epsom salts will even alleviate the pain of corns. Epsom salts are available at your local pharmacy.

Treatment: Add two tablespoons of Epsom salts to a basin of warm water. Soak feet for 15 minutes, advises podiatrist Andrew Schink, D.P.M, of Eugene, Oregon, a former president of the Oregon Podiatric Medical Association. Afterward, pat your feet dry and apply a moisturizing cream or lotion.

FEVERFEW

If you suffer from debilitating migraines, feverfew is the remedy you've been waiting for. Feverfew is an herb well known for its ability to fight migraine headaches. Apparently the herb inhibits blood-vessel dilation, a factor that plays a major role in causing migraine headaches.

Fortunately, you can grow your own feverfew indoors or out. (If you live on a farm with a ready supply of manure, use the manure to enrich the soil.) For best results, sow the feverfew seedlings in late spring.

Treatment: For migraine control, chew two fresh (or frozen) feverfew leaves a day, or take a capsule containing 85 milligrams of leaf material. Feverfew is quite bitter. Most people prefer the capsules to chewing the leaves.

ICE CREAM HEADACHES

Enjoying the occasional dish of ice cream is fine, but be careful not to eat it too quickly. Eating ice cream too fast can give you a headache. The pain can actually begin within 60 seconds of the first bite; it can last from several seconds to a minute or more.

Joseph Hulihan, M.D., a neurologist at Temple University Hospital in Philadelphia, says no one knows for sure why consuming a frozen dessert—and sometimes a cold drink—can trigger headaches in some people. He theorizes that the sudden change in temperature overstimulates the nervous system and causes the headache reaction. Migraine sufferers are among those who are particularly likely to experience ice cream headaches because of their sensitivity to temperature changes.

If feverfew capsules do not provide relief after a few weeks, don't give up on the herb without changing brands. A recent study showed some brands of feverfew capsules contain only trace amounts of the herb.

Warning: Talk to your doctor before using feverfew for the treatment of migraine headaches. Do not take feverfew if you are using an anti-clotting medication such as warfarin. Feverfew may cause sores inside the mouth. If it does, discontinue taking the herb. If you are pregnant, do not use this herb without first consulting your doctor.

FOLIC ACID

Whether you get folic acid in your food or in tablet form, make sure you do, in fact, get it—and in the right amounts—especially if you're a woman.

Folic acid is a B vitamin that helps the body form protein, stomach acid, and a blood component called hemoglobin. Research shows folic acid can help reduce the risk of cervical cancer, prevent anemia and sprue (impaired absorption of nutrients in the intestine), and reduce the risk that a woman will have a child with birth defects. The U.S. Centers for Disease Control (CDC) in Atlanta recently reported that if all women of childbearing age consumed the right amounts of folic acid, 50 to 70 percent of all brain and spinal cord defects present at birth could be prevented.

Folic acid also helps protect against heart disease—in men as well as women—as indicated in a study by the Canadian health agency Health Canada. The study found that individuals with low levels of folic acid in their blood increased their risk of developing fatal heart disease by 69 percent.

Treatment: If you are pregnant, take 0.6 milligrams of folic acid a day. (The U.S. government recommends 0.4 milligrams, but recent studies indicate 0.6 milligrams might offer more protection. Ask your physician which amount is right for you.) If you are not pregnant, you need to take at least 0.18 milligrams of folic acid a day.

Among foods rich in folic acid are broccoli, beans, lettuce, spinach, peas, lentils, tomatoes, potatoes, cantaloupe, orange juice, whole-grain cereals, whole-wheat bread, and liver. Be careful how you prepare the vegetables. Overcooking can diminish their nutritional value. You can also supplement your diet by taking folic acid tablets, which are available over the counter at your local pharmacy.

Warning: Although taking large amounts of folic acid can eliminate the symptoms of anemia, the illness may still remain. It's always wise, therefore, to see your physician if you develop anemia or have symptoms of anemia (fatigue, shortness of breath, headaches, dizziness, weakness, and faintness).

GARLIC

An herb of the lily family, garlic's healing reputation is almost as powerful as its smell. Not only does this wonder herb seem to prevent infection by the influenza virus, but garlic may work on the cold front, too.

Some research suggests that garlic may also reduce blood pressure and cholesterol levels and thin the blood, reducing the risk of blood clots. (Blood clots are a major cause of heart attacks and stroke.) In particular, there are two ingredients in garlic that produce this lifesaving, blood-thinning effect: adenosine and allicin.

Treatment: Adenosine remains effective even after cooking, according to studies by researchers at the University of Heidelberg in Germany. Allicin is effective only when garlic is eaten raw. So, if you're watching your heart's health, it's best to eat raw garlic—despite what your neighbors say.

To treat colds and flu, researchers recommend amounts of between six to 12 cloves of garlic a day. To help reduce blood pressure, cholesterol, and the likelihood of clots, three to ten cloves of garlic a day are recommended.

Warning: Talk to your doctor before taking higher than recommended doses of garlic, however. Garlic causes stomach upset in

No More Nausea

Feeling a little nauseous? Frequent nausea sufferers are gaining relief from their symptoms thanks to a wristband that delivers a mild electric current. The band transmits the current to the same spot on the wrist that acupuncturists zero in on when treating nausea. The electric current apparently blocks nausea signals sent to the brain.

Kenneth Koch, M.D., a gastroenterologist at Hershey Medical Center in Hershey, Pennsylvania, reported that almost 75 percent of his patients who use the wristband have found relief from chronic nausea. Among persons being helped by the wristband are those suffering from motion sickness and morning sickness, as well as those suffering from nausea as a result of chemotherapy.

some people. If you are pregnant, do not use large amounts of this herb without first consulting your physician.

GINGER

Ever since ancient Asian sailors chewed ginger to quell their queasy stomachs, people have been using this re-markable spice to relieve stomach upset and nausea. So if your tummy is giving you trouble or you're suf-fering from a bout of motion sickness, why not give ginger a try?

Treatment: For motion sickness, the recommended dose is 1,500 milligrams of ginger in capsule form ap-proximately 30 minutes before travel. (You can drink a 12-ounce glass of ginger ale instead, but it will be less effective against some of the more intense symptoms.)

To relieve mild stomach distress, drink ginger ale or use ginger tea. To make gin-ger tea, use 2 teaspoons of powdered or grated ginger root per cup of boiling water. Steep 10 minutes before drinking.

Warning: If you are pregnant, do not use this herb without first consulting your doctor. Ginger has been shown to cause heartburn in some people.

MINERAL OIL

Mineral oil is an excellent remedy for relieving dry skin and psoriasis. Psoriasis is a disorder that is thought to be caused by an overproduction of skin cells. If you have the condition, your skin cells mature and turn over in a brisk three or four days instead of the usual 28 or 30 days. The skin thickens and turns into red bumps covered by silvery scales, often on the the arms, ears, scalp, and pubic area.

For psoriasis sufferers, one of the advantages of mineral oil—besides the fact that it is an inexpensive substitute for costly moisturizers—is that it is pure, containing no additives or perfumes that could further irritate the skin.

Treatment: For psoriasis sufferers, the National Psoriasis Foundation recommends that you bathe first to moisten the skin. The mineral oil should be applied afterward, acting as a sealant to lock in the moisture. To treat simple dry-skin problems, apply mineral oil directly to affected areas as needed.

Warning: Although some dictionaries define mineral oil as a laxative, most doctors frown on using it to relieve constipation because it interferes with the body's absorption of vitamins. If you take mineral oil as a laxative, follow your physician's instructions exactly.

THUMBS DOWN

Does your child suck on her thumb? In babies and young children, thumbsucking is a normal, soothing reflex. As the permanent teeth come in, however, continued thumbsucking can misalign teeth and cause improper growth of the mouth. According to the American Dental Association:

- At the latest, children should stop thumbsucking by the time the permanent teeth come in, usually around six or seven years of age.
- Parents should reward the child when he or she refrains from thumbsucking.
- Parents can bandage the child's thumb at night or place a sock over the child's hand to prevent thumbsucking during sleep.
- Talk to your dentist about other methods that may help your child break the habit.

OIL OF CLOVES

If you have a toothache and can't see your dentist immediately, use oil of cloves in the meantime to help soothe the soreness.

The oil—which is distilled from the flower buds of a tropical evergreen tree—is a medically approved remedy that can bring immediate relief. But be careful. The active ingredient in the oil, eugenol, is so powerful that it can damage the nerve of your tooth if you apply it at full strength.

At your local pharmacy, you can buy full-strength oil of cloves or pre-mixed preparations that contain eugenol.

Treatment: Use diluted oil of cloves or a preparation containing eugenol. If you buy a eugenol preparation, follow the instructions on the label. If you buy full-strength oil of cloves, make a mixture containing equal parts of clove oil and olive oil. Then dip a ball of cotton into the mixture and apply it to the tooth. You may feel a sting for ten seconds or so. Use oil of cloves as needed until you see your dentist.

Warning: Do not use undiluted clove oil and do not use clove oil as a replacement for dental treatment. It is a pain reliever, not a healer. As a rule, you should not use oil of cloves for more than a week. If you are pregnant, do not use oil of cloves without first consulting your doctor.

PARSLEY

If you'd like to try a natural remedy for bad breath, chew some parsley. The chlorophyll it contains, once digested, will sweeten the air you exhale, making you a pleasure to be around. Chlorophyll is the active ingredient in many commercial breath fresheners.

No, parsley won't cure bad breath, but it will help mask it. So, if you don't like commercial mouthwashes, it makes good "scents" to try this perennial herb.

Treatment: To freshen breath, eating a few sprigs of parsley will usually suffice.

Warning: High doses of parsley oil have been shown to cause headache, nausea, vertigo, hives, and liver and kidney damage. If you are pregnant, do not use parsley oil without first consulting your doctor.

PEPPERMINT

Menthol, the oil distilled from peppermint and other mints, is used to flavor beverages, desserts, candy, chewing gum, and medicine. The U.S. Food and Drug Administration (FDA) has approved menthol as an active ingredient for several over-the-counter indigestion remedies because of the mint's ability to relax stomach muscles. So, for occasional indigestion, you might want to give peppermint tea a try.

Treatment: Boil 1 or 2 teaspoons of dried or fresh, crushed peppermint leaves to make peppermint tea. Drink a cup of the tea two or three times a day to help relieve symptoms of indigestion.

Warning: Avoid taking peppermint if you suffer frequent bouts of heartburn. Peppermint relaxes the stomach muscles, which could allow backup of stomach contents. Do not give peppermint to babies or small children. The menthol in the tea may cause a choking sensation. Do not take peppermint if you are breast-feeding; peppermint can reduce milk flow.

ROSEMARY

Can rosemary really improve memory, prevent baldness, control dandruff, heal canker sores, lower blood pressure, strengthen blood vessels, aid digestion, dispel intestinal gas, relieve headaches, and alleviate the symptoms of arthritis and earaches?

There is some evidence that this evergreen shrub of the mint family can do some of these things. But, as is the case with so many herbs, the evidence is far from conclusive.

But rosemary might be worth a try if you're a bit on edge. Rosemary has been shown throughout history to be effective in calming nerves and cheering dampened spirits.

Treatment: To make a rosemary tea, add a teaspoon of crushed rosemary leaves to a cup of boiling water and steep for approximately 10 minutes. Drink 2 or 3 cups a day.

Warning: If your anxiety is constant or severe, see your physician. If you are pregnant, do not take this herb without first consulting your doctor.

SALT CAPSULES

Many of you know the feeling: You're kneeling in the garden, pulling weeds. When you rise suddenly, you feel dizzy and a little faint.

Some people actually lose consciousness and fall. Elderly folks and underweight young people are among those at high risk of suffering fainting spells that occur as a result of suddenly rising from a chair, a bed, or the floor.

Why do such spells occur?

When you stand up quickly, gravity pulls blood downward, reducing the flow of blood—and its life-giving cargo, oxygen—to the brain. Without enough oxygen, the brain "goes to sleep" momentarily and you black out and fall. As you lie there, gravity no longer pulls blood downward and, in a few moments, normal blood flow is restored and you become conscious again. If you suffer frequent or occasional fainting spells, taking salt tablets could help you. But before you try this therapy, you should see your physician.

Here's why:

An underlying problem—such as a heartbeat abnormality or heart disease—could be causing the problem. You could also have low blood sugar. However, if your physician finds that you have no serious health problems, including high blood pressure—then you might want to try salt therapy.

Salt expands the volume of blood plasma, which in turn improves circulation. In studies at the University of Leeds in England, researchers found that people who suffered from fainting spells benefited from taking daily salt capsules. After two months, 70 percent of the participants in the study said they could stand up suddenly without feeling faint.

Wishwa N. Kapoor, M.D., chief of general medicine at the University of Pittsburgh, gives patients who suffer from fainting spells 3 to 6 grams of salt a day. Substantial dosages are necessary, he says, to achieve the desired result.

Treatment: If your physician approves, take salt capsules to prevent fainting spells. Ask your doctor to recommend a dosage. (Your physician may recommend that you simply increase your dietary salt intake instead of taking salt tablets.)

SALT WATER

In ancient times, salt was highly valued as a seasoning and preservative agent. Roman soldiers received it as a form of pay. In fact, our modern word "salary" is derived from the Latin word "salerium," which referred to the soldiers' salt allotment.

Today salt remains highly valuable to civilization. If you doubt this, try to find a canned or packaged food that doesn't contain it. And try to find a medical book that doesn't discuss its importance in the makeup of various therapeutic solutions.

Salt water can be used to relieve many minor ills, including nasal congestion and sore throat.

Treatment: Here's how to use salt water to soothe some common ailments:

- *Nasal congestion.* When you have a respiratory infection such as a cold or the flu, molecules called cytokines cause the inside of your nose to become swollen and inflamed. Salt water can help remedy inflammation and reduce mucus production.

  Stephen R. Jones, M.D., of Good Samaritan Hospital in Portland, Oregon, recommends making a salt-water spray. First, add a teaspoon of salt to a quart of water to make the solution. Then fill a nasal-spray bottle with the solution and spray three times into each nostril. Repeat about five times a day.

- *Sore throat and hoarseness.* Add a teaspoon of salt to a glass of warm water. Gargle the solution and

DUST MITES

Wash your clothes regularly in hot water. Otherwise, they could become nesting places for dust mites that cause allergic reactions, including asthma attacks. Researchers have long known that mites tend to set up housekeeping in sheets, pillow cases, and other bedding. But a study at the University of Sydney in Australia revealed that dust mites inhabit clothing as well. The researchers found that one of every two garments harbored enough dust mites to cause an allergic reaction in some people.

What attracts the mites to clothing is food: They feed on dead skin cells. To kill the mites, wash your clothes in water with a temperature of more than 130° F. Hard-to-wash items (children's toys, pillows) can be placed in a freezer until frozen—the low temperatures can also kill mites.

then spit it out. Repeat this procedure every two hours or so.

- *Gingivitis.* This condition inflames and swells the gums and causes bleeding. If uncorrected, it could lead to tooth loss. If you notice signs of gingivitis, make an appointment to see your dentist. In the meantime, rinse your mouth with salt water (1 teaspoon to a glass of warm water) to soothe the gums and help wash away the bacteria that cause gingivitis. Simply roll the water around in your mouth for 30 seconds or so, then spit it out.

SITZ BATH

Many medical experts agree that sitting in a sitz bath of warm water is one of the best ways to relieve the pain and swelling of hemorrhoids.

A sitz bath is a bathtub in the shape of a chair. When you sit on it, only your buttocks and hips are immersed. If you don't have a sitz bath, your bathtub will do. Sitting in the warm water will help relieve the pain of hemorrhoids and increase blood flow to the area to reduce swollen veins.

Treatment: First, make certain your bathtub or sitz bath is clean. Next, run in enough warm water to bathe your hemorrhoids. (In a bathtub, you'll need only about four inches of water.) Sit in the water with your knees raised. If the hard surface of the tub floor bothers you, try sitting on an inflatable "doughnut" available at many pharmacies.

ST. JOHN'S WORT

St. John's wort is one herb that continues to live up to its centuries-old reputation as a remedy for depression. In a recent study involving 1,757 patients, doctors at Ludwig Maximilians University in Munich, Germany, found that St. John's wort was as effective as antidepressant drugs in relieving the symptoms of mild to moderately severe depression. St. John's wort also caused fewer side effects than traditional antidepressant medications. The herb contains several chemical compounds responsible for its depression-fighting power.

Information is lacking on how St. John's wort affects the severely depressed, however. Similarly, no information has been provided on the long-term effects of St. John's wort in regard to delayed side effects and preventing depression relapse.

Should you try it? In view of the significant evidence in its favor, you may want to explore the possibility if you suffer from depression. Talk with your physician about using the herb, and arrive at a decision together.

Treatment: To make an infusion, use 1 to 2 teaspoons of dried herb per cup of boiling water. Steep 10 to 15 minutes. Drink up to three cups a day.

Warning: If you are suffering from depression, see your physician. St. John's wort should not be taken in large amounts without your doctor's approval. While using St. John's wort, do not take amphetamines, narcotics, the amino acids tryptophan and tyrosine, diet pills, asthma inhalants, nasal decongestants, or cold or hay fever medication. In addition, don't drink beer, wine, or coffee, or eat salami, yogurt, chocolate, fava beans, or smoked or pickled items. If St. John's wort causes headache, stiff neck, or nausea, use less of the herb or stop using it altogether. If these side effects persist, consult your doctor immediately. If you are pregnant, do not use this herb without first consulting your doctor.

SYRUP OF IPECAC

Your medicine chest isn't complete if it doesn't contain a bottle of syrup of ipecac. This remedy is used to induce vomiting in those who have swallowed a non-caustic poison.

Before using syrup of ipecac, call an ambulance and your local poison-control center (usually based at a hospital) for emergency assistance. Report the type of poison ingested, if known, and any other information the control center requests. (If the individual swallowed medication, be prepared to read the label on the container to emergency personnel.) If the control center advises using syrup of ipecac—for example, to bring up drugs or poisonous plants—proceed with treatment.

Syrup of ipecac should not be used for all poisoning emergencies. In particular, you should not induce vomiting with syrup of ipecac, or any other remedy, if the patient is unconscious; if you don't know what kind of poison the patient swallowed; or if the patient has swallowed a caustic poison. Caustic poisons—such as lye, bleach, paint thinner, turpentine, and gasoline—burn when they are swallowed. Forcing the patient to vomit a caustic poison could seriously damage tissue when the poison comes back up.

Treatment: Give children 1 tablespoon of syrup of ipecac and adults two tablespoons. Children should drink half a glass of water afterward, and adults should drink a full glass of water or more. Vomiting should occur within 20 minutes. If it doesn't, repeat the dosage.

Individuals who are conscious and who have swallowed a caustic poison should be given milk, water, or milk of magnesia (a tablespoon in a cup of water) to dilute the poison. Seek medical attention immediately.

Warning: If you suspect poisoning, call an ambulance and your local poison-control center immediately. Do not induce vomiting unless directed to do so by emergency personnel.

TEA BAG

To rid yourself of those tiny ulcerations of the mouth called canker sores, grab a tea bag. Tea contains an astringent called tannic acid, which causes skin cells to shrink.

Treatment: To obtain relief from the pain of canker sores, apply the wet tea bag directly to the canker sore and hold in place for a few minutes.

WITCH HAZEL

Witch hazel is a woody shrub of eastern North America that bears yellow flowers. Witch hazel lotion has long been recognized as an effective treatment for a variety of conditions. An ingredient in it, catechol tannin, acts as an astringent, constricting capillaries and thereby reducing irritation and swelling.

Witch hazel leaves, twigs, and bark contain fairly high concentrations of tannins which can reduce irritation and swelling. Oil extracted from the bark is mixed with alcohol to make a soothing lotion.

The herb's cooling, astringent action can be used to treat a variety of external conditions, including cuts, burns and sunburn, scalds, bruises, inflammations, and hemorrhoids. Witch hazel is also recommended as a gargle for sore throats and sores in the mouth. (Commercial witch hazel water may not contain tannins, but it does contain other chemicals with reported antiseptic, anesthetic, astringent, and anti-inflammatory action.)

Treatment: For an astringent decoction, boil 1 teaspoon of powdered leaves or twigs per cup of water for 10 minutes. Strain and cool. Apply the decoction directly to the skin or mix into an ointment. To make a gargle, use 1 teaspoon of bark per cup of boiling water. Steep 10 minutes and strain.

Warning: Do not eat or drink witch hazel. The herb is meant to be used as a topical application only. If witch hazel causes minor discomforts, such as skin irritation, dilute the solution or stop using it. Let your doctor know if you experience unpleasant side effects or if your symptoms do not improve within two weeks. See your doctor if you are suffering from serious sunburn. If you are pregnant, do not use witch hazel without first consulting your doctor.

YARROW POULTICE

The yarrow herb can be found in pastures and along roadsides throughout the northern hemisphere. Native Americans and pioneers applied it to minor skin cuts and abrasions to help fight infection.

Treatment: Yarrow can be used to promote healing in several ways. To make a poultice, bring water to a boil and pour the boiling water over the yarrow flowers, completely immersing them. Place the flowers in a strainer to drain excess water. Wrap the flowers in gauze and apply the poultice after thoroughly washing the affected area. (Do not apply yarrow to unwashed cuts. Because yarrow works fast, it will stop the bleeding while sealing in dirt.) Remove the poultice and apply a bandage after the bleeding subsides.

You can also place ground-up yarrow tips in a cup of hot water. Mix in glycerin, boric acid, and oil of wintergreen (a few teaspoons of each). Apply the resulting semi-liquid mixture to the injury site and wrap it in gauze.

A third option is to sprinkle yarrow powder on the cut. You can buy yarrow powder at natural-food stores.

Warning: Do not ingest yarrow. The herb is meant to be used as a topical application only. If you are pregnant, do not use this herb without first consulting your doctor.

Index   157

Index   159